BARIATRIC WEIGHT-LOSS JOURNAL

BARIATRIC
WEIGHT-LOSS
JOURNAL

A DAILY FOOD TRACKER
FOR BEFORE AND AFTER SURGERY

ROCKRIDGE
PRESS

For general information on our other products and services or to obtain technical support, please contact our Customer Care Department within the United States at (866) 744-2665, or outside the United States at (510) 253-0500.

Rockridge Press publishes its books in a variety of electronic and print formats. Some content that appears in print may not be available in electronic books, and vice versa.

Interior and Cover Designer: Irene Vandervoort
Art Producer: Sara Feinstein
Editor: Leah Zarra
Production Editor: Jax Berman
Production Manager: Martin Worthington

Illustration used under license from Shutterstock

Paperback ISBN: 978-1-63878-935-2
R0

CONTENTS

INTRODUCTION vii

PART I
Getting Started I
Bariatric Weight-Loss Basics 2

Nutritional Know-How 3

Additional Tips for Success 7

How to Use This Journal 8

PART 2
Preparing for Bariatric Surgery 13
The Pre-Op Diet 14

Setting a Baseline 18

Mental Preparation 18

Home Preparation 19

The Day Of 20

Going Home 21

PART 3
Your Post–Bariatric Surgery Weight-Loss Journal 23

INTRODUCTION

Bariatric surgery refers to a few highly effective procedures used to achieve and maintain significant weight loss. Bariatric procedures can have a tremendous positive impact on health conditions, sometimes almost immediately.

This journal will help guide you through what happens before and after bariatric surgery. Part 1 will outline the basics of bariatric surgery. Part 2 will help prepare you during the two weeks leading up to surgery. Part 3 will then track what you're eating after surgery from day 1 until day 224 (eight months).

In parts 1 and 2, you will find ideas and tips for dietary and lifestyle adjustments that will prepare you for surgery and life after. The big key to post-op success is a lifelong commitment to following nutritional guidelines and building healthy habits. Tracking your progress in part 3 will help you achieve success both physically and mentally; it will get you healthier and not just thinner.

There will likely be many celebrations and challenges throughout this process, and, as you know, success doesn't happen overnight. Start each morning with a fresh perspective, and focus on working toward small goals each day.

Now, let's get to it!

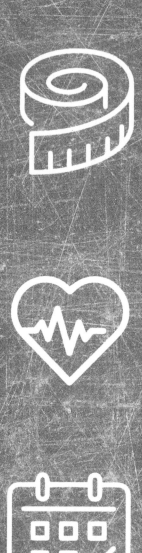

PART 1

Getting Started

In this part, we'll cover all the essentials you need to know to begin the journey to bariatric surgery. You'll learn about the key aspects of nutrition that will help you establish healthy habits.

Bariatric Weight-Loss Basics

Congratulations on your decision to have weight-loss surgery! This is an exciting chance to reset your mind, body, and lifestyle. Even with extensive knowledge about the procedure, surgery and the required lifestyle changes can be overwhelming. But surgery seemed like a necessary step toward better control of your health, and your medical team agreed. This journal will help allay any fears and give you the tools you need to embrace your new lifestyle.

Throughout your journey, you'll notice that small, sustainable changes will have the biggest impact on your life and health. But you can get there, one step at a time, with hard work and dedication.

Rather than thinking about how far you are from where you want to be, consider what you can do right now. For example, if your goal is to become more active, consider taking the stairs instead of the elevator, or getting off the bus before your usual stop to walk the rest of the way. If your goal is to improve your dietary choices, consider skipping the starchy side dish and adding extra vegetables to your plate. Much like taking a shower or brushing your teeth, these small decisions will become daily habits as you practice them.

TYPES OF BARIATRIC SURGERY

The most common bariatric surgeries today are the Roux-en-Y gastric bypass (RYGB), laparoscopic sleeve gastrectomy (LSG), and adjustable gastric band (AGB). All bariatric surgeries work to reduce hunger and encourage portion control, and some surgeries work at an even deeper metabolic level. Some surgeries also have been shown to improve type 2 diabetes, high blood pressure, sleep apnea, fatty liver, and other comorbidities. Determining which procedure is best for you will require the expertise of your surgeon and medical team. Each surgery has its own advantages and disadvantages, but they all help you take control of your health.

ROUX-EN-Y GASTRIC BYPASS is commonly known as gastric bypass, and this procedure is considered the "gold standard" of weight-loss surgery. It is reversible, restricts stomach capacity, and favorably alters gut hormones, but it requires the longest hospital stays associated with bariatric sugery and has higher surgical complication rates.

LAPAROSCOPIC SLEEVE GASTRECTOMY patients will have about 80 percent of their stomachs removed under the care of their surgical teams. The procedure works by significantly limiting the amount of food the stomach can hold at a time—only a small, tubular pouch the shape of a banana remains. But its greatest effect is on gut hormones that impact hunger, satiety, and blood sugar control. There is a risk of developing long-term vitamin and mineral deficiencies as well as acid reflux.

ADJUSTABLE GASTRIC BAND procedures insert an inflatable band near the top of the stomach to create a small stomach pouch. The size of the pouch can be reduced gradually over time, by filling the band with saline via a port underneath the abdominal wall. Increasing the tightness of the band in this way affects how easily food can move from the small pouch into the lower stomach. The pouch is designed to limit hunger and promote a feeling of fullness.

Nutritional Know-How

You don't need to be a nutrition expert to understand and follow a bariatric eating plan. Let's review the principles for eating after surgery.

LIQUIDS

Staying hydrated after surgery is the first and most important rule. Drinking enough liquids will not only increase your energy, but also help significantly with your weight loss. Additionally, dehydration is the most common complication after bariatric surgery and one that can easily be prevented. It can be challenging at first, partly because you cannot drink with meals or 30 minutes before or after eating. Be proactive and always carry a beverage with you. Focus on drinking small amounts throughout the morning and afternoon to prevent trying to catch up later—and remember that your smaller stomach will prohibit you from chugging large amounts of fluid at one time.

WHAT TO DRINK: Water, milk, soy milk, protein shakes, and decaffeinated tea or coffee (without added cream or sugar)

AMOUNT PER DAY: 64 to 100 ounces, progressing in volume throughout your post-op diet stages

WHAT TO LIMIT OR AVOID: Juices, caffeinated beverages (including soda, coffee, tea, and energy drinks), carbonated beverages, alcohol, lemonade, sweetened tea, sports drinks, and any sugar-sweetened beverages

PROTEIN

Protein is the building block of muscle and tissue and the most important macronutrient to take in after your surgery. It's crucial to eat adequate protein while following a very low-calorie diet. When you eat enough protein, you will feel energized, lose more fat while preserving muscle, and experience longer post-meal satisfaction. After your surgery, it will initially seem like you are taking in only water and protein-rich foods. As you progress, you will slowly add more mixed meals into your diet.

WHAT TO EAT: Eggs, poultry (chicken and turkey without skin, lean nitrate-free chicken or turkey sausage, ground chicken and turkey breast), all fish and seafood, low-fat or nonfat dairy products (low-fat Greek yogurt, 1% or nonfat cottage cheese, 1% or nonfat milk and cheese), lean beef (if tolerated) beginning three months post-op (sirloin, loin, round roast or steak, and lean or supreme lean ground beef), lean pork (if tolerated) beginning three months post-op (tenderloin, top loin chop, and ham with visible fat removed), and vegetarian protein sources (beans, nuts, lentils, and seeds)

AMOUNT PER DAY: 60 to 100 grams

WHAT TO LIMIT OR AVOID: High-fat dairy products (cream and whole milk), high-fat cuts of beef or pork (pork sausage, bacon, bologna, salami, pork ribs, and ground beef), and skin-on poultry

CARBOHYDRATES

During the initial post-op diet, you will take in few to no carbs. Carbohydrates can be found in two varieties: simple or complex. Simple carbohydrates are digested quickly and easily turn into sugar in our blood, giving us an energy rush and subsequent crash. Simple carbs include foods made with white refined flour, candies, juice drinks, and many processed foods. Complex carbo-hydrates are digested more slowly and are rich in fiber, vitamins, and minerals. They include 100 percent whole-grain foods, fruits, and vegetables. Focus on limiting simple carbs and eating more complex carbs.

WHAT TO EAT: Fresh fruits, vegetables, potatoes with skin, oat-meal, 100 percent whole-grain bread products (toasted is better tolerated than doughy fresh), brown or wild rice or 100 percent whole wheat pasta (if tolerated), and barley and ancient grains (quinoa, spelt, farro, millet)

AMOUNT PER DAY: Very small amounts initially; after the first year and over the long term, aim for 35 to 45 percent total calories from carbohydrates

WHAT TO LIMIT OR AVOID: Any white refined grain products (white bread, white pasta, and crackers), cookies, candies, cakes, pastries, and chips

FATS

Dietary fats are important to absorb the essential fat-soluble vitamins A, D, E, and K. Additionally, there are some essential fatty acids (omega-3s and omega-6s) our bodies cannot make and that must be ingested.

Be cautious with processed foods labeled as fat-free or low-fat, because the fat is often replaced with excessive sugar or sodium to improve the flavor. Dairy products, particularly milk, yogurt, and cottage cheese, should be eaten in low-fat or nonfat form to save on calories and artery-clogging saturated fats.

Choose full-fat foods in the form of vegetable oils, nuts, seeds, avocados, olives, and fatty fish—all of which are heart healthy.

WHAT TO EAT: Avocado, chia seeds, fatty fish (salmon, mackerel, and tuna), other seafood and shellfish, flaxseed, extra-virgin olive oil, almonds, walnuts, peanuts, and all-natural nut butters

AMOUNT PER DAY: Very limited amounts initially; over the long term, no more than 30 percent of your total calories should be from fats (mostly healthy versions and less than 7 percent from saturated fats)

WHAT TO LIMIT: Butter, tropical oils (palm and coconut oil), full-fat dairy, and miscellaneous vegetable oils

WHAT TO AVOID: Animal fats (fat on meats, lard), fried foods, trans fats, and foods high in processed saturated fats

VITAMIN AND MINERAL SUPPLEMENTS

Food is the best source of nutrients for your body after surgery. However, because of the restricted amount of food you'll be able to eat, all bariatric surgery patients need to take vitamin and mineral supplements. Follow the recommendations from your bariatric surgery team for specific details, but here are some general recommendations.

TAKE YOUR VITAMINS AS CLOSE TO MEALTIME AS POSSIBLE. Some vitamins are best absorbed when accompanied by food. It's okay to break the rule of "no liquids with meals" to take just a few sips to get your pills down if you are taking a capsule or tablet version.

AVOID USING GUMMY VITAMINS POST-OP. Most versions are high in sugar and calories and do not meet the 100 to 200 percent recommended daily allowance. If you find a version that meets your nutritional needs, verify it first with your medical team to make sure it's approved for you.

LOOK FOR SUPPLEMENTS WITH THE USP VERIFIED SYMBOL. Because herbal supplements and vitamins are not regulated by the FDA, this symbol lets you know you are getting a high-quality brand. You may choose to purchase specialty vitamins such as Bariatric Advantage or Celebrate that are targeted to weight-loss surgery patients. Keep in mind that specialty supplements are expensive, and they aren't necessary if you choose the proper over-the-counter equivalents.

Additional Tips for Success

While the bariatric surgery will certainly jump start your weight-loss journey, there are a few other tips to set you up for success. You'll see that the daily entries in this journal provide space to track your water intake, sleep, and exercise.

SLEEP: Poor sleep can result in increased appetite and weight gain, which in turn makes it harder to sleep going forward. Additionally, your body needs rest to heal after surgery. Aim for six to eight hours of sleep per night.

EXERCISE: Exercise is a great companion to bariatric surgery, seeing as the goal is to be healthier, not just lose weight. After surgery, start taking short walks or slow jogs for 15 minutes every other day. Introduce or reintroduce other exercises as your body heals to help build strength and improve your quality of life. No matter what you do, try to do a little more every couple weeks to start building strength.

Try to incorporate a new healthy habit every month, and use the notes section every day to track your process.

How to Use This Journal

This journal will help you along your weight-loss journey through daily, weekly, and monthly reporting and reflection. Journals are a valuable tool for navigating life after bariatric surgery, because there's so much to track. Using a journal also increases your awareness of your lifestyle choices and habits by giving you room to write down what you're eating, monitor your intake of macros, note how you feel after consuming different foods, and make informed, conscious decisions for the next day and week ahead.

DAILY AND WEEKLY ENTRIES

For each week, there will be a four-page spread of seven daily entries to log meals and associated macros, water intake, exercise, mood, and sleep. Space is included for you to write your breakfast, lunch, dinner, and snacks consumed every day. A sample daily entry appears on page 9.

When completing the entries, here are some helpful tips:

- Include the food quantity, even if just a quick estimate such as "handful of nuts."

- Complete your log after every meal, glass of water, or activity so you don't miss anything.

- Jot down notes throughout the day on how you're feeling, particularly if you notice any mood changes or drops in energy.

At the beginning of each week, you'll find intention questions to prepare for the week and create action steps. Use these questions to get excited for the coming week and to revisit your goals, such as hitting your macros.

SAMPLE DAILY ENTRY

DAY 15 Date: _October 19_		Mood Check: 😊 🙂 😐 🙁 ☹️
BREAKFAST	**LUNCH**	**Water:**
9 am	12 pm	🥤🥤🥤🥤🥤 🥤🥛🥛🥛🥛
1 soft scrambled egg	1/2 cup Lemon-Dijon tuna salad	**Sleep (Hours):**
Proteins:16 g Carbs:10 g Fats:10 g	Proteins:25 g Carbs:12 g Fats:12 g	8
DINNER	**SNACKS**	**Exercise Type:**
6 pm	3 pm /8 pm	Walking
3/4 cup Split pea soup	10 almonds 1/4 cup low-fat Greek yogurt	**Exercise (Minutes):**
Proteins:25 g Carbs:11 g Fats:13 g	Proteins:24 g Carbs:10 g Fats:10 g	30
DAILY MACROS Proteins: 35 % Carbs: 25 % Fats: 40 %		

Notes: Exercised in the morning and felt the endorphins all day. Try to space out my water consumption tomorrow so I can drink eight glasses of water.

FOUR-WEEK CHECK-IN

At the start of the journal, you'll find a chart to log your initial weight and body measurements for your upper arms, chest, waist, hips, thighs, and calves. Here are some tips for where (and how) to measure:

- Upper arms: Bend your elbow. Flex your arm and measure your bicep.

- Chest: Measure the widest part around your bust or chest.

- Waist: Measure the narrowest part of your torso.

- Hips: Measure the widest part of your glutes (your butt muscle).

- Thighs: Measure the midpoint between the lower glutes and the back of your knee.

- Calves: Measure halfway between your knee and your ankle.

- When weighing and measuring yourself, remember to always do it at the same time of day (morning is usually best) and in the same way for the most consistent and pre-cise numbers.

Every four weeks, there will be a check-in with the same chart to assess your progress on your weight-loss goals. This chart will also include an additional column to note your progress (decreases, no change, or increases). Beneath each chart is a series of questions to reflect on your progress and set new goals.

Though you can check your own progress at more frequent intervals, this journal uses four-week increments for more accurate measurements. Your weight fluctuates from day to day, so measuring over a longer time span will give you more realistic results.

10/8/22

Neck 15.71 in

Chest/Bust 48.66 in

Waist 46.81 in

Hips 55.72 in

Biceps R 16.49 L 16.84

Thigh R 30.15 L 30.66

Calves R 19.09 L 19.81

Waist to Hip Ratio .84

Weight 258.5

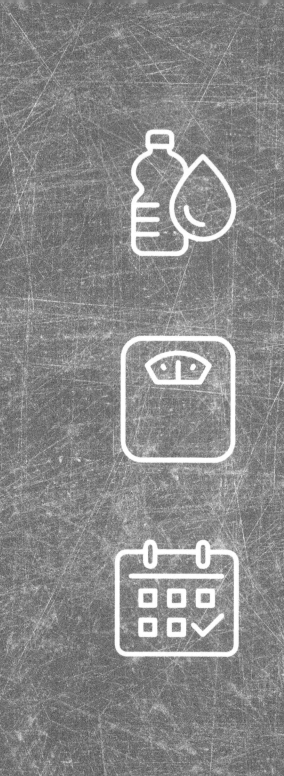

PART 2

Preparing for Bariatric Surgery

This part of the journal will act as a guide to prepare you for your bariatric surgery. We'll cover some presurgical basics, as well as set your presurgical baseline. Presurgical check-lists will help make the day of surgery as easy as possible.

The Pre-Op Diet

Prior to surgery, most patients are required to follow a pre-op diet to lose weight and reduce the amount of fat in and around the liver and abdomen. Your exact pre-op guidelines and any required weight-loss goal will be determined by your surgical team, but this section offers general guidance for the preoperative phase, which will also guide you into post-op living.

GUIDELINES FOR THE PRE-OP DIET

Pre-op guidelines vary among clinics and are sometimes patient-specific. You will likely be required to follow a low-calorie, low-carbohydrate, or liquid diet for at least two weeks prior to surgery.

PROTEIN SHAKES AND SUPPLEMENTS

If you are having bariatric surgery, you will at some point use protein shakes or powders. Protein strengthens and protects muscle tissue and encourages your body to burn fat instead of muscle. If you are required to follow a liquid diet before surgery, protein shakes are a great meal-replacement option.

Here are a few recommendations for protein supplements to get you started:

- Whey protein isolate: Lactose-free, milk-based, complete protein (best tolerated and most absorbable for bariatric patients)

- Soy protein: Plant-based, complete protein

- Egg white protein: Non-milk-based, complete protein

- Whey protein concentrate: Milk-based, complete protein containing lactose (may cause discomfort for gastric bypass patients with lactose intolerance after surgery)

FAT

Prior to surgery, you will need to be mindful about the amount and type of fat you consume to gain control over your caloric intake and help you lose weight. Pay close attention to your fat intake, and read labels to identify hidden sources of fat.

WHAT TO EAT

- Almonds
- Avocados
- Canola oil
- Chia seeds
- Fatty fish (such as salmon, tuna, and mackerel)
- Flaxseed
- Nut butters, all-natural
- Olive oil
- Olives
- Peanuts
- Seafood
- Walnuts

WHAT TO LIMIT

- Animal fats
- Baked goods
- Chips
- Chocolate
- Cream sauces
- Foods high in saturated fat
- Fried foods
- Full-fat dairy products
- High-fat condiments such as mayonnaise
- High-fat salad dressings
- Stick margarines containing hydrogenated oils
- Tropical oils

SUGAR

Sugar is an especially sneaky ingredient that you'll find in almost every prepared food you buy. Some foods that are unexpectedly high in sugar include ketchup, yogurt, dried fruit, barbecue and other sauces, fruit juices, pasta sauce, flavored coffees, sports drinks, premade soups, frozen dinners, granola bars, protein bars, and even some protein shakes.

HIGH-CARB FOODS

Reducing your carbohydrate intake has been shown to improve blood sugar control, help manage cravings, and aid in weight loss. While it may not be necessary to go completely carb-free before surgery, it's a good opportunity to make some adjustments.

WHAT TO EAT

- Dairy products, low-fat
- Nuts
- Seeds

- Vegetables, non-starchy (like asparagus, broccoli, cauliflower, kale, onions, spinach, and zucchini)
- Whole fruits

WHAT TO AVOID

- Chips
- Corn
- Dried fruit
- Flour, white (as in breads, crackers, pasta, and tortillas)

- Fried foods
- Potatoes
- Rice
- Sweet sauces and dressings

DRINKS

Prior to surgery, aim for at least 48 to 64 ounces of hydrating fluids per day. Avoid beverages high in fat or sugar, and try to limit your caffeine intake. After surgery, you may find it difficult to stay hydrated due to the inability to drink with meals or consume large amounts of fluid quickly.

WHAT TO DRINK

- Broth, low-sodium
- Sports drinks, sugar-free
- Tea, unsweetened

- Water
- Water, flavored, sugar-free
- Water, infused

WHAT TO AVOID

- Alcohol
- Coffee

- Fruit juices
- Sodas and other carbonated drinks

HABITS TO AVOID

Prior to surgery, you will be asked to quit smoking and using tobacco. Both can delay healing and increase your risk for blood clots, pneumonia, and ulcers. You will also be asked to abstain from alcohol for a period before and after surgery.

Setting a Baseline

Tracking your mood and diet before surgery will help you establish a solid baseline to refer to.

The first two weeks of trackers and check-in at the beginning of part 3 are meant to help you see the progress you make from month to month. Take the time to fill out every page, and get into the habit of tracking your food, exercise, sleep, water intake, and mood so it's easy to maintain after surgery.

Mental Preparation

After attending seminars, appointments, classes, and more, you are ready to move forward, and your care team agrees. As you approach your surgery date, it is completely normal to feel a mixture of excitement and nervousness. Here are some tips to help calm your mind and body:

- Practice taking slow, deep breaths.

- Practice mindful meditation techniques or listen to a guided meditation.

- Practice progressive muscle relaxation by slowly tensing and relaxing each muscle group in your body, beginning with your toes and moving up to your jaw.

- Use guided-imagery techniques to visualize yourself in a place that brings you comfort, joy, and calmness.

- Take a walk and get some fresh air.

- Listen to your favorite soothing music.

- Talk to a loved one about your thoughts and feelings.

Write down your thoughts leading up to surgery. Do you feel ready, excited, nervous? What steps have you taken to prepare?

_____

_____

_____

_____

_____

Home Preparation

Focusing on why you're having surgery and the results you are most excited about achieving is an excellent way to prepare your mind. For additional peace of mind, having your post-op supplies ready before your surgery will also help you feel confident and equipped for the journey ahead.

HOME KITCHEN CHECKLIST:

☐ Measuring cups

☐ Hydrating fluids

☐ Protein shakes

☐ A reusable water bottle

☐ A blender or blender bottles

☐ Small bowls and plates

☐ Small airtight storage containers

☐ Appetizer spoons and forks

☐ A mug warmer (to keep small plates warm)

☐ Recommended vitamin and mineral supplements

☐ A food scale

☐ An insulated bag or cooler

The Day Of

The day of your surgery is the first day of the rest of your life. Your mind, body, and home are prepared for the next steps. Trust in yourself and your ability to achieve your goals. Life after surgery will not always be easy, but your hard work and dedication will pay off. You've got this!

The day of your surgery, keep in mind the following:

- You will likely be expected to avoid drinking any fluids for at least four hours before your procedure.

- Once you are awake following surgery, you will likely be encouraged to drink slowly. Your stomach will only be able to hold a small amount of fluid, so it may take you over an hour to drink eight ounces of water.

- You will likely experience some discomfort with gas trapped in your abdomen. Stand up and walk around as often as you can to alleviate some of this pain.

Take note of how you're feeling the day of your surgery. Remind yourself of your health goals and why you began this journey.

_____

_____

_____

_____

_____

_____

_____

_____

WHAT TO PACK

- [ ] Any medications or necessary medical equipment
- [ ] A pillow to hold against your abdomen on the ride home
- [ ] Comfortable, loose-fitting clothing
- [ ] Slippers or house socks
- [ ] Any toiletries
- [ ] Mouthwash
- [ ] Lip balm
- [ ] Unscented lotion
- [ ] Unscented deodorant
- [ ] Earplugs or noise-canceling headphones
- [ ] Chargers for your personal electronics
- [ ] Protein shakes

Going Home

After surgery, you may feel a bit groggy and may experience some nausea, gas pains, and tenderness near your abdominal incision sites. Your medical team may also encourage you to begin walking to relieve gas pain and prevent blood clots. Depending on your procedure, you will likely spend one to three days in the hospital.

Prior to discharge, make sure to review your post-op guidelines with your surgical team. Discuss medication requirements and clarify when to start your post-op vitamin and mineral supplements. Additionally, make sure you have scheduled your post-op follow-up appointments and that you have information on how to contact someone with questions or concerns.

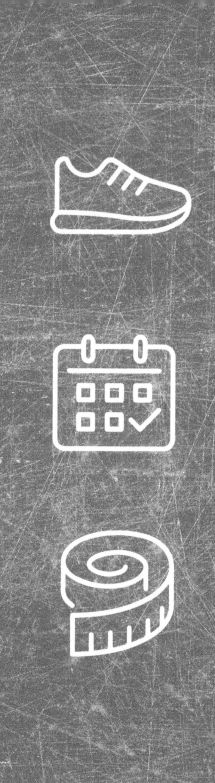

PART 3

Your Post-
Bariatric Surgery
Weight-Loss Journal

Welcome to part 3: your post-surgery weight-loss journal! For the next eight months, these pages will help you record your daily, weekly, and monthly numbers and progress. Remember that weight loss is different for every person, so use this journal to celebrate your achievements at your pace.

BASELINE CHECK-IN

MEASUREMENT	CURRENT
WEIGHT (LB)	
UPPER ARMS (IN)	
CHEST (IN)	
WAIST (IN)	
HIPS (IN)	
THIGHS (IN)	
CALVES (IN)	

CONGRATULATIONS ON STARTING YOUR JOURNEY!

What are you most proud of today?

_____

_____

_____

What was your biggest challenge leading up to the surgery?

_____

_____

_____

What are some goals you would like to work toward for the next four weeks?

_____

_____

_____

Reflect on your mood over the past month. Did you notice differences related to your eating habits?

_____

_____

_____

WEEKLY INTENTION

What are you excited about for this week?

Proteins: _____ %
Carbs: _____ %
Fats: _____ %

_____

_____

_____

_____

What is something you'd like to work on this week? _____

_____

_____

_____

DAY I	Date: _____	Mood Check: 😃 🙂 😐 🙁 ☹️
BREAKFAST	**LUNCH**	Water:
		Sleep (Hours):
Proteins: ___ g Carbs: ___ g Fats: ___ g	Proteins: ___ g Carbs: ___ g Fats: ___ g	_____
DINNER	**SNACKS**	Exercise Type: _____ Exercise (Minutes):
Proteins: ___ g Carbs: ___ g Fats: ___ g	Proteins: ___ g Carbs: ___ g Fats: ___ g	
DAILY MACROS Proteins: ___ % Carbs: ___ % Fats: ___ %		_____

Notes:

DAY 2   Date: _____   Mood Check: 😃 🙂 😐 🙁 ☹️

BREAKFAST	LUNCH	Water:
		🥛🥛🥛🥛 🥛🥛🥛🥛
		Sleep (Hours):
Proteins: ___ g Carbs: ___ g Fats: ___ g	Proteins: ___ g Carbs: ___ g Fats: ___ g	_____
DINNER	SNACKS	Exercise Type: _____ Exercise (Minutes):
Proteins: ___ g Carbs: ___ g Fats: ___ g	Proteins: ___ g Carbs: ___ g Fats: ___ g	_____
DAILY MACROS Proteins: ___ % Carbs: ___ % Fats: ___ %		

Notes:

DAY 3   Date: _____   Mood Check: 😃 🙂 😐 🙁 ☹️

BREAKFAST	LUNCH	Water:
		🥛🥛🥛🥛 🥛🥛🥛🥛
		Sleep (Hours):
Proteins: ___ g Carbs: ___ g Fats: ___ g	Proteins: ___ g Carbs: ___ g Fats: ___ g	_____
DINNER	SNACKS	Exercise Type: _____ Exercise (Minutes):
Proteins: ___ g Carbs: ___ g Fats: ___ g	Proteins: ___ g Carbs: ___ g Fats: ___ g	_____
DAILY MACROS Proteins: ___ % Carbs: ___ % Fats: ___ %		

Notes:

DAY 4

Date: _____ Mood Check: 😃 🙂 😐 🙁 😣

BREAKFAST	LUNCH	Water:
		🥤🥤🥤🥤 🥤🥤🥤🥤
		Sleep (Hours):
Proteins: ___g Carbs: ___g Fats: ___g	Proteins: ___g Carbs: ___g Fats: ___g	_____

DINNER	SNACKS	Exercise Type:
		_____
		Exercise (Minutes):
Proteins: ___g Carbs: ___g Fats: ___g	Proteins: ___g Carbs: ___g Fats: ___g	_____

DAILY MACROS   Proteins: ___%   Carbs: ___%   Fats: ___%

Notes:

DAY 5

Date: _____ Mood Check: 😃 🙂 😐 🙁 😣

BREAKFAST	LUNCH	Water:
		🥤🥤🥤🥤 🥤🥤🥤🥤
		Sleep (Hours):
Proteins: ___g Carbs: ___g Fats: ___g	Proteins: ___g Carbs: ___g Fats: ___g	_____

DINNER	SNACKS	Exercise Type:
		_____
		Exercise (Minutes):
Proteins: ___g Carbs: ___g Fats: ___g	Proteins: ___g Carbs: ___g Fats: ___g	_____

DAILY MACROS   Proteins: ___%   Carbs: ___%   Fats: ___%

Notes:

DAY 6   Date: _____   Mood Check: 😀 🙂 😐 🙁 ☹️

BREAKFAST	LUNCH	Water:
		🥛🥛🥛🥛 🥛🥛🥛🥛
		Sleep (Hours):
Proteins: ___ g Carbs: ___ g Fats: ___ g	Proteins: ___ g Carbs: ___ g Fats: ___ g	_____
DINNER	**SNACKS**	Exercise Type:
		_____
		Exercise (Minutes):
Proteins: ___ g Carbs: ___ g Fats: ___ g	Proteins: ___ g Carbs: ___ g Fats: ___ g	
DAILY MACROS Proteins: ___ % Carbs: ___ % Fats: ___ %		_____

Notes:

DAY 7   Date: _____   Mood Check: 😀 🙂 😐 🙁 ☹️

BREAKFAST	LUNCH	Water:
		🥛🥛🥛🥛 🥛🥛🥛🥛
		Sleep (Hours):
Proteins: ___ g Carbs: ___ g Fats: ___ g	Proteins: ___ g Carbs: ___ g Fats: ___ g	_____
DINNER	**SNACKS**	Exercise Type:
		_____
		Exercise (Minutes):
Proteins: ___ g Carbs: ___ g Fats: ___ g	Proteins: ___ g Carbs: ___ g Fats: ___ g	
DAILY MACROS Proteins: ___ % Carbs: ___ % Fats: ___ %		_____

Notes:

WEEKLY INTENTION

TARGET MACROS

What are you excited about for this week?

Proteins: _____ %
Carbs: _____ %
Fats: _____ %

_____

_____

_____

_____

What is something you'd like to work on this week? _____

_____

_____

_____

DAY 8 Date: _____		Mood Check: ☺ ☺ 😐 ☹ ☹
BREAKFAST	**LUNCH**	Water:
		🥛🥛🥛🥛🥛 🥛🥛🥛🥛🥛
		Sleep (Hours):
Proteins: __ g Carbs: __ g Fats: __ g	Proteins: __ g Carbs: __ g Fats: __ g	_____
DINNER	**SNACKS**	Exercise Type:
		_____
		Exercise (Minutes):
Proteins: __ g Carbs: __ g Fats: __ g	Proteins: __ g Carbs: __ g Fats: __ g	_____
DAILY MACROS Proteins: __ % Carbs: __ % Fats: __ %		

Notes:

DAY 9   Date: _____   Mood Check: 😀 🙂 😐 🙁 ☹️

BREAKFAST	LUNCH	Water:
		🥤🥤🥤🥤 🥤🥤🥤🥤
		Sleep (Hours):
Proteins: ___ g Carbs: ___ g Fats: ___ g	Proteins: ___ g Carbs: ___ g Fats: ___ g	_____
DINNER	**SNACKS**	Exercise Type:
		_____
		Exercise (Minutes):
Proteins: ___ g Carbs: ___ g Fats: ___ g	Proteins: ___ g Carbs: ___ g Fats: ___ g	_____
DAILY MACROS Proteins: ___ % Carbs: ___ % Fats: ___ %		

Notes:

DAY 10   Date: _____   Mood Check: 😀 🙂 😐 🙁 ☹️

BREAKFAST	LUNCH	Water:
		🥤🥤🥤🥤 🥤🥤🥤🥤
		Sleep (Hours):
Proteins: ___ g Carbs: ___ g Fats: ___ g	Proteins: ___ g Carbs: ___ g Fats: ___ g	_____
DINNER	**SNACKS**	Exercise Type:
		_____
		Exercise (Minutes):
Proteins: ___ g Carbs: ___ g Fats: ___ g	Proteins: ___ g Carbs: ___ g Fats: ___ g	_____
DAILY MACROS Proteins: ___ % Carbs: ___ % Fats: ___ %		

Notes:

WEEK 2

DAY 11   Date: _____   Mood Check: 😀 🙂 😐 🙁 ☹️

BREAKFAST	LUNCH	Water:
		🥤🥤🥤🥤🥤 🥤🥤🥤🥤🥤
		Sleep (Hours):
Proteins: ___ g Carbs: ___ g Fats: ___ g	Proteins: ___ g Carbs: ___ g Fats: ___ g	_____
DINNER	SNACKS	Exercise Type:
		_____
		Exercise (Minutes):
Proteins: ___ g Carbs: ___ g Fats: ___ g	Proteins: ___ g Carbs: ___ g Fats: ___ g	_____
DAILY MACROS Proteins: ___ % Carbs: ___ % Fats: ___ %		

Notes:

DAY 12   Date: _____   Mood Check: 😀 🙂 😐 🙁 ☹️

BREAKFAST	LUNCH	Water:
		🥤🥤🥤🥤🥤 🥤🥤🥤🥤🥤
		Sleep (Hours):
Proteins: ___ g Carbs: ___ g Fats: ___ g	Proteins: ___ g Carbs: ___ g Fats: ___ g	_____
DINNER	SNACKS	Exercise Type:
		_____
		Exercise (Minutes):
Proteins: ___ g Carbs: ___ g Fats: ___ g	Proteins: ___ g Carbs: ___ g Fats: ___ g	_____
DAILY MACROS Proteins: ___ % Carbs: ___ % Fats: ___ %		

Notes:

DAY 13 Date: _____ Mood Check: ☺ ☺ ☺ ☹ ☹

BREAKFAST	LUNCH	Water:
		🥤🥤🥤🥤 🥤🥤🥤🥤
		Sleep (Hours):
Proteins: ___ g Carbs: ___ g Fats: ___ g	Proteins: ___ g Carbs: ___ g Fats: ___ g	_____
DINNER	**SNACKS**	Exercise Type:
		_____
		Exercise (Minutes):
Proteins: ___ g Carbs: ___ g Fats: ___ g	Proteins: ___ g Carbs: ___ g Fats: ___ g	_____
DAILY MACROS Proteins: ___ % Carbs: ___ % Fats: ___ %		

Notes:

DAY 14 Date: _____ Mood Check: ☺ ☺ ☺ ☹ ☹

BREAKFAST	LUNCH	Water:
		🥤🥤🥤🥤 🥤🥤🥤🥤
		Sleep (Hours):
Proteins: ___ g Carbs: ___ g Fats: ___ g	Proteins: ___ g Carbs: ___ g Fats: ___ g	_____
DINNER	**SNACKS**	Exercise Type:
		_____
		Exercise (Minutes):
Proteins: ___ g Carbs: ___ g Fats: ___ g	Proteins: ___ g Carbs: ___ g Fats: ___ g	_____
DAILY MACROS Proteins: ___ % Carbs: ___ % Fats: ___ %		

Notes:

WEEKLY INTENTION

What are you excited about for this week?

Proteins: _____ %
Carbs: _____ %
Fats: _____ %

_____

_____

_____

_____

What is something you'd like to work on this week? _____

_____

_____

_____

DAY 15	Date: _____	Mood Check: ☺ ☺ ☺ ☹ ☹

BREAKFAST	LUNCH	Water:
		🥤🥤🥤🥤 🥤🥤🥤🥤
		Sleep (Hours):
Proteins: ___ g Carbs: ___ g Fats: ___ g	Proteins: ___ g Carbs: ___ g Fats: ___ g	
DINNER	SNACKS	Exercise Type:
		Exercise (Minutes):
Proteins: ___ g Carbs: ___ g Fats: ___ g	Proteins: ___ g Carbs: ___ g Fats: ___ g	
DAILY MACROS Proteins: ___ % Carbs: ___ % Fats: ___ %		

Notes:

DAY 16   Date: _____   Mood Check: 😃 🙂 😐 🙁 😞

BREAKFAST	LUNCH	Water:
		🥛🥛🥛🥛 🥛🥛🥛🥛
		Sleep (Hours):
Proteins: ___ g Carbs: ___ g Fats: ___ g	Proteins: ___ g Carbs: ___ g Fats: ___ g	_____
DINNER	SNACKS	Exercise Type:
		_____
		Exercise (Minutes):
Proteins: ___ g Carbs: ___ g Fats: ___ g	Proteins: ___ g Carbs: ___ g Fats: ___ g	_____
DAILY MACROS Proteins: ___ % Carbs: ___ % Fats: ___ %		

Notes:

DAY 17   Date: _____   Mood Check: 😃 🙂 😐 🙁 😞

BREAKFAST	LUNCH	Water:
		🥛🥛🥛🥛 🥛🥛🥛🥛
		Sleep (Hours):
Proteins: ___ g Carbs: ___ g Fats: ___ g	Proteins: ___ g Carbs: ___ g Fats: ___ g	_____
DINNER	SNACKS	Exercise Type:
		_____
		Exercise (Minutes):
Proteins: ___ g Carbs: ___ g Fats: ___ g	Proteins: ___ g Carbs: ___ g Fats: ___ g	_____
DAILY MACROS Proteins: ___ % Carbs: ___ % Fats: ___ %		

Notes:

DAY 18　Date: _____　Mood Check: 😃 🙂 😐 🙁 😞

BREAKFAST	LUNCH	Water:
		🥛🥛🥛🥛 🥛🥛🥛🥛
		Sleep (Hours):
Proteins: ___ g Carbs: ___ g Fats: ___ g	Proteins: ___ g Carbs: ___ g Fats: ___ g	_____
DINNER	**SNACKS**	Exercise Type:
		_____
		Exercise (Minutes):
Proteins: ___ g Carbs: ___ g Fats: ___ g	Proteins: ___ g Carbs: ___ g Fats: ___ g	_____
DAILY MACROS　Proteins: ___ %　Carbs: ___ %　Fats: ___ %		

Notes:

DAY 19　Date: _____　Mood Check: 😃 🙂 😐 🙁 😞

BREAKFAST	LUNCH	Water:
		🥛🥛🥛🥛 🥛🥛🥛🥛
		Sleep (Hours):
Proteins: ___ g Carbs: ___ g Fats: ___ g	Proteins: ___ g Carbs: ___ g Fats: ___ g	_____
DINNER	**SNACKS**	Exercise Type:
		_____
		Exercise (Minutes):
Proteins: ___ g Carbs: ___ g Fats: ___ g	Proteins: ___ g Carbs: ___ g Fats: ___ g	_____
DAILY MACROS　Proteins: ___ %　Carbs: ___ %　Fats: ___ %		

Notes:

DAY 20   Date: _____   Mood Check: 😀 😊 😐 🙁 😣

BREAKFAST	LUNCH	Water:
		🥛🥛🥛🥛 🥛🥛🥛🥛
		Sleep (Hours):
Proteins: ___ g Carbs: ___ g Fats: ___ g	Proteins: ___ g Carbs: ___ g Fats: ___ g	_____
DINNER	**SNACKS**	Exercise Type: _____
		Exercise (Minutes):
Proteins: ___ g Carbs: ___ g Fats: ___ g	Proteins: ___ g Carbs: ___ g Fats: ___ g	
DAILY MACROS Proteins: ___ % Carbs: ___ % Fats: ___ %		_____

Notes:

DAY 21   Date: _____   Mood Check: 😀 😊 😐 🙁 😣

BREAKFAST	LUNCH	Water:
		🥛🥛🥛🥛 🥛🥛🥛🥛
		Sleep (Hours):
Proteins: ___ g Carbs: ___ g Fats: ___ g	Proteins: ___ g Carbs: ___ g Fats: ___ g	_____
DINNER	**SNACKS**	Exercise Type: _____
		Exercise (Minutes):
Proteins: ___ g Carbs: ___ g Fats: ___ g	Proteins: ___ g Carbs: ___ g Fats: ___ g	
DAILY MACROS Proteins: ___ % Carbs: ___ % Fats: ___ %		_____

Notes:

WEEKLY INTENTION

What are you excited about for this week?

Proteins: _____ %
Carbs: _____ %
Fats: _____ %

_____

_____

_____

_____

What is something you'd like to work on this week? _____

_____

_____

_____

DAY 22	Date: _____	Mood Check: 😃 🙂 😐 🙁 ☹️
BREAKFAST	**LUNCH**	Water:
		🥛🥛🥛🥛🥛 🥛🥛🥛🥛🥛
		Sleep (Hours):
Proteins: ___ g Carbs: ___ g Fats: ___ g	Proteins: ___ g Carbs: ___ g Fats: ___ g	_____
DINNER	**SNACKS**	Exercise Type:
		_____
		Exercise (Minutes):
Proteins: ___ g Carbs: ___ g Fats: ___ g	Proteins: ___ g Carbs: ___ g Fats: ___ g	
DAILY MACROS Proteins: ___ % Carbs: ___ % Fats: ___ %		_____

Notes:

DAY 23 Date: _____ Mood Check: ☺ ☺ ☺ ☹ ☹

BREAKFAST	LUNCH	Water:
		🥤🥤🥤🥤 🥤🥤🥤🥤
		Sleep (Hours):
Proteins: ___ g Carbs: ___ g Fats: ___ g	Proteins: ___ g Carbs: ___ g Fats: ___ g	_____
DINNER	**SNACKS**	Exercise Type:
		_____
		Exercise (Minutes):
Proteins: ___ g Carbs: ___ g Fats: ___ g	Proteins: ___ g Carbs: ___ g Fats: ___ g	_____
DAILY MACROS Proteins: ___ % Carbs: ___ % Fats: ___ %		

Notes:

DAY 24 Date: _____ Mood Check: ☺ ☺ ☺ ☹ ☹

BREAKFAST	LUNCH	Water:
		🥤🥤🥤🥤 🥤🥤🥤🥤
		Sleep (Hours):
Proteins: ___ g Carbs: ___ g Fats: ___ g	Proteins: ___ g Carbs: ___ g Fats: ___ g	_____
DINNER	**SNACKS**	Exercise Type:
		_____
		Exercise (Minutes):
Proteins: ___ g Carbs: ___ g Fats: ___ g	Proteins: ___ g Carbs: ___ g Fats: ___ g	_____
DAILY MACROS Proteins: ___ % Carbs: ___ % Fats: ___ %		

Notes:

DAY 25 | Date: _____ Mood Check: 😃 🙂 😐 🙁 ☹️

BREAKFAST	LUNCH	Water:
		🥛🥛🥛🥛 🥛🥛🥛🥛
		Sleep (Hours):
Proteins: ___ g Carbs: ___ g Fats: ___ g	Proteins: ___ g Carbs: ___ g Fats: ___ g	_____
DINNER	**SNACKS**	Exercise Type:
		_____
		Exercise (Minutes):
Proteins: ___ g Carbs: ___ g Fats: ___ g	Proteins: ___ g Carbs: ___ g Fats: ___ g	_____
DAILY MACROS	Proteins: ___ % Carbs: ___ % Fats: ___ %	

Notes:

DAY 26 | Date: _____ Mood Check: 😃 🙂 😐 🙁 ☹️

BREAKFAST	LUNCH	Water:
		🥛🥛🥛🥛 🥛🥛🥛🥛
		Sleep (Hours):
Proteins: ___ g Carbs: ___ g Fats: ___ g	Proteins: ___ g Carbs: ___ g Fats: ___ g	_____
DINNER	**SNACKS**	Exercise Type:
		_____
		Exercise (Minutes):
Proteins: ___ g Carbs: ___ g Fats: ___ g	Proteins: ___ g Carbs: ___ g Fats: ___ g	_____
DAILY MACROS	Proteins: ___ % Carbs: ___ % Fats: ___ %	

Notes:

DAY 27

Date: _____   Mood Check: ☺ ☺ 😐 🙁 ☹

BREAKFAST	LUNCH	Water:
		🥛🥛🥛🥛🥛 🥛🥛🥛🥛🥛
		Sleep (Hours):
Proteins: ___ g Carbs: ___ g Fats: ___ g	Proteins: ___ g Carbs: ___ g Fats: ___ g	_____
DINNER	**SNACKS**	Exercise Type:
		_____
		Exercise (Minutes):
Proteins: ___ g Carbs: ___ g Fats: ___ g	Proteins: ___ g Carbs: ___ g Fats: ___ g	_____
DAILY MACROS Proteins: ___ % Carbs: ___ % Fats: ___ %		

Notes:

DAY 28

Date: _____   Mood Check: ☺ ☺ 😐 🙁 ☹

BREAKFAST	LUNCH	Water:
		🥛🥛🥛🥛🥛 🥛🥛🥛🥛🥛
		Sleep (Hours):
Proteins: ___ g Carbs: ___ g Fats: ___ g	Proteins: ___ g Carbs: ___ g Fats: ___ g	_____
DINNER	**SNACKS**	Exercise Type:
		_____
		Exercise (Minutes):
Proteins: ___ g Carbs: ___ g Fats: ___ g	Proteins: ___ g Carbs: ___ g Fats: ___ g	_____
DAILY MACROS Proteins: ___ % Carbs: ___ % Fats: ___ %		

Notes:

FOUR-WEEK CHECK-IN

Date: _____

MEASUREMENT	CURRENT	MONTH CHANGE
WEIGHT (LB)		
UPPER ARMS (IN)		
CHEST (IN)		
WAIST (IN)		
HIPS (IN)		
THIGHS (IN)		
CALVES (IN)		

CONGRATULATIONS ON MAKING IT THIS FAR!

What are you most proud of accomplishing in the past four weeks?

_____

_____

_____

_____

What was your biggest challenge over the past four weeks?

_____

_____

_____

_____

_____

What are some goals you would like to work toward for the next four weeks?

_____

_____

_____

_____

Reflect on your mood over the past month. Did you notice differences related to your eating habits?

_____

_____

_____

_____

_____

WEEKLY INTENTION

What are you excited about for this week?

Proteins: _____ %
Carbs: _____ %
Fats: _____ %

_____

_____

_____

_____

What is something you'd like to work on this week? _____

_____

_____

_____

DAY 29	Date: _____	Mood Check: 😃 🙂 😐 🙁 ☹️
BREAKFAST	**LUNCH**	Water:
		Sleep (Hours):
Proteins: ___ g Carbs: ___ g Fats: ___ g	Proteins: ___ g Carbs: ___ g Fats: ___ g	_____
DINNER	**SNACKS**	Exercise Type: _____
		Exercise (Minutes):
Proteins: ___ g Carbs: ___ g Fats: ___ g	Proteins: ___ g Carbs: ___ g Fats: ___ g	_____
DAILY MACROS	Proteins: ___ % Carbs: ___ % Fats: ___ %	

Notes:

DAY 30   Date: _____   Mood Check: 😀 🙂 😐 🙁 ☹️

BREAKFAST	LUNCH	Water:
		🥤🥤🥤🥤 🥤🥤🥤🥤
		Sleep (Hours):
Proteins: ___ g Carbs: ___ g Fats: ___ g	Proteins: ___ g Carbs: ___ g Fats: ___ g	_____
DINNER	**SNACKS**	Exercise Type:
		_____
		Exercise (Minutes):
Proteins: ___ g Carbs: ___ g Fats: ___ g	Proteins: ___ g Carbs: ___ g Fats: ___ g	_____
DAILY MACROS Proteins: ___ % Carbs: ___ % Fats: ___ %		

Notes:

DAY 31   Date: _____   Mood Check: 😀 🙂 😐 🙁 ☹️

BREAKFAST	LUNCH	Water:
		🥤🥤🥤🥤 🥤🥤🥤🥤
		Sleep (Hours):
Proteins: ___ g Carbs: ___ g Fats: ___ g	Proteins: ___ g Carbs: ___ g Fats: ___ g	_____
DINNER	**SNACKS**	Exercise Type:
		_____
		Exercise (Minutes):
Proteins: ___ g Carbs: ___ g Fats: ___ g	Proteins: ___ g Carbs: ___ g Fats: ___ g	_____
DAILY MACROS Proteins: ___ % Carbs: ___ % Fats: ___ %		

Notes:

DAY 32   Date: _____   Mood Check: 😀 🙂 😐 🙁 😣

BREAKFAST	LUNCH	Water:
		🥤🥤🥤🥤 🥤🥤🥤🥤
		Sleep (Hours):
Proteins: ___ g Carbs: ___ g Fats: ___ g	Proteins: ___ g Carbs: ___ g Fats: ___ g	_____
DINNER	**SNACKS**	Exercise Type:
		_____
		Exercise (Minutes):
Proteins: ___ g Carbs: ___ g Fats: ___ g	Proteins: ___ g Carbs: ___ g Fats: ___ g	_____
DAILY MACROS Proteins: ___ % Carbs: ___ % Fats: ___ %		

Notes:

DAY 33   Date: _____   Mood Check: 😀 🙂 😐 🙁 😣

BREAKFAST	LUNCH	Water:
		🥤🥤🥤🥤 🥤🥤🥤🥤
		Sleep (Hours):
Proteins: ___ g Carbs: ___ g Fats: ___ g	Proteins: ___ g Carbs: ___ g Fats: ___ g	_____
DINNER	**SNACKS**	Exercise Type:
		_____
		Exercise (Minutes):
Proteins: ___ g Carbs: ___ g Fats: ___ g	Proteins: ___ g Carbs: ___ g Fats: ___ g	_____
DAILY MACROS Proteins: ___ % Carbs: ___ % Fats: ___ %		

Notes:

DAY 34   Date: _____   Mood Check: 😃 🙂 😐 🙁 😣

BREAKFAST	LUNCH	Water:
		🥛🥛🥛🥛🥛 🥛🥛🥛🥛🥛
		Sleep (Hours):
Proteins: ___ g Carbs: ___ g Fats: ___ g	Proteins: ___ g Carbs: ___ g Fats: ___ g	_____
DINNER	**SNACKS**	Exercise Type:
		_____
		Exercise (Minutes):
Proteins: ___ g Carbs: ___ g Fats: ___ g	Proteins: ___ g Carbs: ___ g Fats: ___ g	_____
DAILY MACROS Proteins: ___ % Carbs: ___ % Fats: ___ %		

Notes:

DAY 35   Date: _____   Mood Check: 😃 🙂 😐 🙁 😣

BREAKFAST	LUNCH	Water:
		🥛🥛🥛🥛🥛 🥛🥛🥛🥛🥛
		Sleep (Hours):
Proteins: ___ g Carbs: ___ g Fats: ___ g	Proteins: ___ g Carbs: ___ g Fats: ___ g	_____
DINNER	**SNACKS**	Exercise Type:
		_____
		Exercise (Minutes):
Proteins: ___ g Carbs: ___ g Fats: ___ g	Proteins: ___ g Carbs: ___ g Fats: ___ g	_____
DAILY MACROS Proteins: ___ % Carbs: ___ % Fats: ___ %		

Notes:

WEEKLY INTENTION

What are you excited about for this week?

Proteins: _____ %
Carbs: _____ %
Fats: _____ %

_____

_____

_____

_____

What is something you'd like to work on this week? _____

_____

_____

_____

DAY 36	Date: _____	Mood Check: ☺ ☺ ☺ ☹ ☹
BREAKFAST	**LUNCH**	Water:
Proteins: ___ g Carbs: ___ g Fats: ___ g	Proteins: ___ g Carbs: ___ g Fats: ___ g	Sleep (Hours): _____
DINNER	**SNACKS**	Exercise Type: _____
		Exercise (Minutes):
Proteins: ___ g Carbs: ___ g Fats: ___ g	Proteins: ___ g Carbs: ___ g Fats: ___ g	_____
DAILY MACROS	Proteins: ___ % Carbs: ___ % Fats: ___ %	

Notes:

DAY 37 Date: _____ Mood Check: 😀 🙂 😐 🙁 ☹️

BREAKFAST	LUNCH	Water:
		🥛🥛🥛🥛 🥛🥛🥛🥛
		Sleep (Hours):
Proteins: ___ g Carbs: ___ g Fats: ___ g	Proteins: ___ g Carbs: ___ g Fats: ___ g	_____
DINNER	SNACKS	Exercise Type:
		_____
		Exercise (Minutes):
Proteins: ___ g Carbs: ___ g Fats: ___ g	Proteins: ___ g Carbs: ___ g Fats: ___ g	_____
DAILY MACROS Proteins: ___ % Carbs: ___ % Fats: ___ %		

Notes:

DAY 38 Date: _____ Mood Check: 😀 🙂 😐 🙁 ☹️

BREAKFAST	LUNCH	Water:
		🥛🥛🥛🥛 🥛🥛🥛🥛
		Sleep (Hours):
Proteins: ___ g Carbs: ___ g Fats: ___ g	Proteins: ___ g Carbs: ___ g Fats: ___ g	_____
DINNER	SNACKS	Exercise Type:
		_____
		Exercise (Minutes):
Proteins: ___ g Carbs: ___ g Fats: ___ g	Proteins: ___ g Carbs: ___ g Fats: ___ g	_____
DAILY MACROS Proteins: ___ % Carbs: ___ % Fats: ___ %		

Notes:

WEEK 6

DAY 39 | Date: _____ Mood Check: 😃 🙂 😐 🙁 ☹️

BREAKFAST	LUNCH	Water:
		🥛🥛🥛🥛 🥛🥛🥛🥛
		Sleep (Hours):
Proteins: __ g Carbs: __ g Fats: __ g	Proteins: __ g Carbs: __ g Fats: __ g	_____
DINNER	**SNACKS**	Exercise Type:
		_____
		Exercise (Minutes):
Proteins: __ g Carbs: __ g Fats: __ g	Proteins: __ g Carbs: __ g Fats: __ g	_____
DAILY MACROS Proteins: __ % Carbs: __ % Fats: __ %		

Notes:

DAY 40 | Date: _____ Mood Check: 😃 🙂 😐 🙁 ☹️

BREAKFAST	LUNCH	Water:
		🥛🥛🥛🥛 🥛🥛🥛🥛
		Sleep (Hours):
Proteins: __ g Carbs: __ g Fats: __ g	Proteins: __ g Carbs: __ g Fats: __ g	_____
DINNER	**SNACKS**	Exercise Type:
		_____
		Exercise (Minutes):
Proteins: __ g Carbs: __ g Fats: __ g	Proteins: __ g Carbs: __ g Fats: __ g	_____
DAILY MACROS Proteins: __ % Carbs: __ % Fats: __ %		

Notes:

DAY 41 Date: _____ Mood Check: 🙂 🙂 😐 🙁 ☹

BREAKFAST	LUNCH	Water:
		🥛🥛🥛🥛🥛 🥛🥛🥛🥛🥛
		Sleep (Hours):
Proteins: ___ g Carbs: ___ g Fats: ___ g	Proteins: ___ g Carbs: ___ g Fats: ___ g	_____
DINNER	SNACKS	Exercise Type:
		_____
		Exercise (Minutes):
Proteins: ___ g Carbs: ___ g Fats: ___ g	Proteins: ___ g Carbs: ___ g Fats: ___ g	
DAILY MACROS Proteins: ___ % Carbs: ___ % Fats: ___ %		_____

Notes:

DAY 42 Date: _____ Mood Check: 🙂 🙂 😐 🙁 ☹

BREAKFAST	LUNCH	Water:
		🥛🥛🥛🥛🥛 🥛🥛🥛🥛🥛
		Sleep (Hours):
Proteins: ___ g Carbs: ___ g Fats: ___ g	Proteins: ___ g Carbs: ___ g Fats: ___ g	_____
DINNER	SNACKS	Exercise Type:
		_____
		Exercise (Minutes):
Proteins: ___ g Carbs: ___ g Fats: ___ g	Proteins: ___ g Carbs: ___ g Fats: ___ g	
DAILY MACROS Proteins: ___ % Carbs: ___ % Fats: ___ %		_____

Notes:

WEEKLY INTENTION

What are you excited about for this week?

Proteins: _____ %
Carbs: _____ %
Fats: _____ %

_____

_____

_____

_____

What is something you'd like to work on this week? _____

_____

_____

_____

DAY 43 Date: _____ Mood Check: 🙂 🙂 😐 😕 ☹️

BREAKFAST	LUNCH	Water:
		🥛🥛🥛🥛🥛 🥛🥛🥛🥛🥛
		Sleep (Hours):
Proteins: __g Carbs: __g Fats: __g	Proteins: __g Carbs: __g Fats: __g	_____
DINNER	SNACKS	Exercise Type:
		_____
		Exercise (Minutes):
Proteins: __g Carbs: __g Fats: __g	Proteins: __g Carbs: __g Fats: __g	_____
DAILY MACROS Proteins: __% Carbs: __% Fats: __%		

Notes:

DAY 44

Date: _____ Mood Check: 😀 😊 😐 😕 😞

BREAKFAST	LUNCH	Water:
		🥛🥛🥛🥛🥛 🥛🥛🥛🥛🥛
		Sleep (Hours):
Proteins: ___ g Carbs: ___ g Fats: ___ g	Proteins: ___ g Carbs: ___ g Fats: ___ g	_____
DINNER	**SNACKS**	Exercise Type: _____
		Exercise (Minutes):
Proteins: ___ g Carbs: ___ g Fats: ___ g	Proteins: ___ g Carbs: ___ g Fats: ___ g	
DAILY MACROS Proteins: ___ % Carbs: ___ % Fats: ___ %		

Notes:

DAY 45

Date: _____ Mood Check: 😀 😊 😐 😕 😞

BREAKFAST	LUNCH	Water:
		🥛🥛🥛🥛🥛 🥛🥛🥛🥛🥛
		Sleep (Hours):
Proteins: ___ g Carbs: ___ g Fats: ___ g	Proteins: ___ g Carbs: ___ g Fats: ___ g	_____
DINNER	**SNACKS**	Exercise Type: _____
		Exercise (Minutes):
Proteins: ___ g Carbs: ___ g Fats: ___ g	Proteins: ___ g Carbs: ___ g Fats: ___ g	
DAILY MACROS Proteins: ___ % Carbs: ___ % Fats: ___ %		

Notes:

WEEK 7

DAY 46 Date: _____ Mood Check: 😀 🙂 😐 🙁 ☹️

BREAKFAST	LUNCH	Water:
		🥤🥤🥤🥤 🥤🥤🥤🥤
		Sleep (Hours):
Proteins: ___ g Carbs: ___ g Fats: ___ g	Proteins: ___ g Carbs: ___ g Fats: ___ g	_____
DINNER	SNACKS	Exercise Type:
		_____
		Exercise (Minutes):
Proteins: ___ g Carbs: ___ g Fats: ___ g	Proteins: ___ g Carbs: ___ g Fats: ___ g	_____
DAILY MACROS Proteins: ___ % Carbs: ___ % Fats: ___ %		

Notes:

DAY 47 Date: _____ Mood Check: 😀 🙂 😐 🙁 ☹️

BREAKFAST	LUNCH	Water:
		🥤🥤🥤🥤 🥤🥤🥤🥤
		Sleep (Hours):
Proteins: ___ g Carbs: ___ g Fats: ___ g	Proteins: ___ g Carbs: ___ g Fats: ___ g	_____
DINNER	SNACKS	Exercise Type:
		_____
		Exercise (Minutes):
Proteins: ___ g Carbs: ___ g Fats: ___ g	Proteins: ___ g Carbs: ___ g Fats: ___ g	_____
DAILY MACROS Proteins: ___ % Carbs: ___ % Fats: ___ %		

Notes:

DAY 48   Date: _____   Mood Check: 😄 😊 😐 🙁 ☹️

BREAKFAST	LUNCH	Water:
		🥤🥤🥤🥤 🥤🥤🥤🥤
		Sleep (Hours):
Proteins: ___ g Carbs: ___ g Fats: ___ g	Proteins: ___ g Carbs: ___ g Fats: ___ g	_____
DINNER	**SNACKS**	Exercise Type:
		_____
		Exercise (Minutes):
Proteins: ___ g Carbs: ___ g Fats: ___ g	Proteins: ___ g Carbs: ___ g Fats: ___ g	_____
DAILY MACROS Proteins: ___ % Carbs: ___ % Fats: ___ %		

Notes:

DAY 49   Date: _____   Mood Check: 😄 😊 😐 🙁 ☹️

BREAKFAST	LUNCH	Water:
		🥤🥤🥤🥤 🥤🥤🥤🥤
		Sleep (Hours):
Proteins: ___ g Carbs: ___ g Fats: ___ g	Proteins: ___ g Carbs: ___ g Fats: ___ g	_____
DINNER	**SNACKS**	Exercise Type:
		_____
		Exercise (Minutes):
Proteins: ___ g Carbs: ___ g Fats: ___ g	Proteins: ___ g Carbs: ___ g Fats: ___ g	_____
DAILY MACROS Proteins: ___ % Carbs: ___ % Fats: ___ %		

Notes:

WEEKLY INTENTION

What are you excited about for this week?

Proteins: _____ %
Carbs: _____ %
Fats: _____ %

_____

_____

_____

What is something you'd like to work on this week? _____

_____

_____

_____

DAY 50	Date: _____	Mood Check: ☺ ☺ ☺ ☹ ☹

BREAKFAST	**LUNCH**	Water:
		🥛🥛🥛🥛🥛 🥛🥛🥛🥛🥛
		Sleep (Hours):
Proteins: ___ g Carbs: ___ g Fats: ___ g	Proteins: ___ g Carbs: ___ g Fats: ___ g	_____
DINNER	**SNACKS**	Exercise Type: _____
		Exercise (Minutes):
Proteins: ___ g Carbs: ___ g Fats: ___ g	Proteins: ___ g Carbs: ___ g Fats: ___ g	_____
DAILY MACROS	Proteins: ___ % Carbs: ___ % Fats: ___ %	

Notes:

DAY 51	Date: _____	Mood Check: 😃 🙂 😐 🙁 😞

BREAKFAST	LUNCH	Water:
		🥤🥤🥤🥤 🥤🥤🥤🥤
		Sleep (Hours):
Proteins: ___ g Carbs: ___ g Fats: ___ g	Proteins: ___ g Carbs: ___ g Fats: ___ g	_____
DINNER	SNACKS	Exercise Type:
		_____
		Exercise (Minutes):
Proteins: ___ g Carbs: ___ g Fats: ___ g	Proteins: ___ g Carbs: ___ g Fats: ___ g	_____
DAILY MACROS	Proteins: ___ % Carbs: ___ % Fats: ___ %	

Notes:

DAY 52	Date: _____	Mood Check: 😃 🙂 😐 🙁 😞

BREAKFAST	LUNCH	Water:
		🥤🥤🥤🥤 🥤🥤🥤🥤
		Sleep (Hours):
Proteins: ___ g Carbs: ___ g Fats: ___ g	Proteins: ___ g Carbs: ___ g Fats: ___ g	_____
DINNER	SNACKS	Exercise Type:
		_____
		Exercise (Minutes):
Proteins: ___ g Carbs: ___ g Fats: ___ g	Proteins: ___ g Carbs: ___ g Fats: ___ g	_____
DAILY MACROS	Proteins: ___ % Carbs: ___ % Fats: ___ %	

Notes:

DAY 53   Date: _____   Mood Check: 😀 🙂 😐 🙁 😣

BREAKFAST	LUNCH	Water:
		🥛🥛🥛🥛 🥛🥛🥛🥛
		Sleep (Hours):
Proteins: ___ g Carbs: ___ g Fats: ___ g	Proteins: ___ g Carbs: ___ g Fats: ___ g	_____
DINNER	SNACKS	Exercise Type:
		_____
		Exercise (Minutes):
Proteins: ___ g Carbs: ___ g Fats: ___ g	Proteins: ___ g Carbs: ___ g Fats: ___ g	_____

DAILY MACROS   Proteins: ___ %   Carbs: ___ %   Fats: ___ %

Notes:

DAY 54   Date: _____   Mood Check: 😀 🙂 😐 🙁 😣

BREAKFAST	LUNCH	Water:
		🥛🥛🥛🥛 🥛🥛🥛🥛
		Sleep (Hours):
Proteins: ___ g Carbs: ___ g Fats: ___ g	Proteins: ___ g Carbs: ___ g Fats: ___ g	_____
DINNER	SNACKS	Exercise Type:
		_____
		Exercise (Minutes):
Proteins: ___ g Carbs: ___ g Fats: ___ g	Proteins: ___ g Carbs: ___ g Fats: ___ g	_____

DAILY MACROS   Proteins: ___ %   Carbs: ___ %   Fats: ___ %

Notes:

DAY 55 Date: _____ Mood Check: 😊 😌 😐 🙁 ☹️

BREAKFAST	LUNCH	Water:
		🥛🥛🥛🥛🥛 🥛🥛🥛🥛🥛
		Sleep (Hours):
Proteins: ___ g Carbs: ___ g Fats: ___ g	Proteins: ___ g Carbs: ___ g Fats: ___ g	_____
DINNER	SNACKS	Exercise Type:
		_____
		Exercise (Minutes):
Proteins: ___ g Carbs: ___ g Fats: ___ g	Proteins: ___ g Carbs: ___ g Fats: ___ g	_____
DAILY MACROS Proteins: ___ % Carbs: ___ % Fats: ___ %		

Notes:

DAY 56 Date: _____ Mood Check: 😊 😌 😐 🙁 ☹️

BREAKFAST	LUNCH	Water:
		🥛🥛🥛🥛🥛 🥛🥛🥛🥛🥛
		Sleep (Hours):
Proteins: ___ g Carbs: ___ g Fats: ___ g	Proteins: ___ g Carbs: ___ g Fats: ___ g	_____
DINNER	SNACKS	Exercise Type:
		_____
		Exercise (Minutes):
Proteins: ___ g Carbs: ___ g Fats: ___ g	Proteins: ___ g Carbs: ___ g Fats: ___ g	_____
DAILY MACROS Proteins: ___ % Carbs: ___ % Fats: ___ %		

Notes:

FOUR-WEEK CHECK-IN

Date: _____

MEASUREMENT	CURRENT	MONTH CHANGE
WEIGHT (LB)		
UPPER ARMS (IN)		
CHEST (IN)		
WAIST (IN)		
HIPS (IN)		
THIGHS (IN)		
CALVES (IN)		

CONGRATULATIONS ON MAKING IT THIS FAR!

What are you most proud of accomplishing in the past four weeks?

_____

_____

_____

_____

What was your biggest challenge over the past four weeks?

_____

_____

_____

_____

_____

What are some goals you would like to work toward for the next four weeks?

_____

_____

_____

_____

_____

Reflect on your mood over the past month. Did you notice differences related to your eating habits?

_____

_____

_____

_____

_____

WEEKLY INTENTION

What are you excited about for this week?

Proteins: _____ %
Carbs: _____ %
Fats: _____ %

_____

_____

_____

_____

What is something you'd like to work on this week? _____

_____

_____

_____

DAY 57	Date: _____		Mood Check: ☺ ☺ ☹ ☹ ☹
BREAKFAST	**LUNCH**		Water:
			Sleep (Hours):
Proteins: ___ g Carbs: ___ g Fats: ___ g	Proteins: ___ g Carbs: ___ g Fats: ___ g		_____
DINNER	**SNACKS**		Exercise Type:
			_____
			Exercise (Minutes):
Proteins: ___ g Carbs: ___ g Fats: ___ g	Proteins: ___ g Carbs: ___ g Fats: ___ g		_____
DAILY MACROS	Proteins: ___ % Carbs: ___ % Fats: ___ %		

Notes:

DAY 58 Date: _____ Mood Check: 😀 😊 😐 🙁 😞

BREAKFAST	LUNCH	Water:
		🥛🥛🥛🥛 🥛🥛🥛🥛
		Sleep (Hours):
Proteins: ___ g Carbs: ___ g Fats: ___ g	Proteins: ___ g Carbs: ___ g Fats: ___ g	_____
DINNER	SNACKS	Exercise Type:
		_____
		Exercise (Minutes):
Proteins: ___ g Carbs: ___ g Fats: ___ g	Proteins: ___ g Carbs: ___ g Fats: ___ g	_____
DAILY MACROS Proteins: ___ % Carbs: ___ % Fats: ___ %		

Notes:

DAY 59 Date: _____ Mood Check: 😀 😊 😐 🙁 😞

BREAKFAST	LUNCH	Water:
		🥛🥛🥛🥛 🥛🥛🥛🥛
		Sleep (Hours):
Proteins: ___ g Carbs: ___ g Fats: ___ g	Proteins: ___ g Carbs: ___ g Fats: ___ g	_____
DINNER	SNACKS	Exercise Type:
		_____
		Exercise (Minutes):
Proteins: ___ g Carbs: ___ g Fats: ___ g	Proteins: ___ g Carbs: ___ g Fats: ___ g	_____
DAILY MACROS Proteins: ___ % Carbs: ___ % Fats: ___ %		

Notes:

DAY 60   Date: _____   Mood Check: 😃 🙂 😐 🙁 😟

BREAKFAST	LUNCH	Water:
		🥤🥤🥤🥤 🥤🥤🥤🥤
		Sleep (Hours):
Proteins: ___ g Carbs: ___ g Fats: ___ g	Proteins: ___ g Carbs: ___ g Fats: ___ g	_____
DINNER	**SNACKS**	Exercise Type:
		_____
		Exercise (Minutes):
Proteins: ___ g Carbs: ___ g Fats: ___ g	Proteins: ___ g Carbs: ___ g Fats: ___ g	_____
DAILY MACROS Proteins: ___ % Carbs: ___ % Fats: ___ %		

Notes:

DAY 61   Date: _____   Mood Check: 😃 🙂 😐 🙁 😟

BREAKFAST	LUNCH	Water:
		🥤🥤🥤🥤 🥤🥤🥤🥤
		Sleep (Hours):
Proteins: ___ g Carbs: ___ g Fats: ___ g	Proteins: ___ g Carbs: ___ g Fats: ___ g	_____
DINNER	**SNACKS**	Exercise Type:
		_____
		Exercise (Minutes):
Proteins: ___ g Carbs: ___ g Fats: ___ g	Proteins: ___ g Carbs: ___ g Fats: ___ g	_____
DAILY MACROS Proteins: ___ % Carbs: ___ % Fats: ___ %		

Notes:

DAY 62   Date: _____   Mood Check: 😀 🙂 😐 🙁 ☹️

BREAKFAST	LUNCH	Water:
		🥛🥛🥛🥛 🥛🥛🥛🥛
		Sleep (Hours):
Proteins: ___ g Carbs: ___ g Fats: ___ g	Proteins: ___ g Carbs: ___ g Fats: ___ g	_____
DINNER	**SNACKS**	Exercise Type:
		_____
		Exercise (Minutes):
Proteins: ___ g Carbs: ___ g Fats: ___ g	Proteins: ___ g Carbs: ___ g Fats: ___ g	_____
DAILY MACROS Proteins: ___ % Carbs: ___ % Fats: ___ %		

Notes:

DAY 63   Date: _____   Mood Check: 😀 🙂 😐 🙁 ☹️

BREAKFAST	LUNCH	Water:
		🥛🥛🥛🥛 🥛🥛🥛🥛
		Sleep (Hours):
Proteins: ___ g Carbs: ___ g Fats: ___ g	Proteins: ___ g Carbs: ___ g Fats: ___ g	_____
DINNER	**SNACKS**	Exercise Type:
		_____
		Exercise (Minutes):
Proteins: ___ g Carbs: ___ g Fats: ___ g	Proteins: ___ g Carbs: ___ g Fats: ___ g	_____
DAILY MACROS Proteins: ___ % Carbs: ___ % Fats: ___ %		

Notes:

WEEKLY INTENTION

What are you excited about for this week?

Proteins: _____ %
Carbs: _____ %
Fats: _____ %

_____

_____

_____

_____

What is something you'd like to work on this week? _____

_____

_____

_____

DAY 64	Date: _____	Mood Check: 😃 🙂 😐 🙁 ☹️
BREAKFAST	**LUNCH**	Water:
		🥛🥛🥛🥛🥛
		🥛🥛🥛🥛🥛
		Sleep (Hours):
Proteins: ___ g Carbs: ___ g Fats: ___ g	Proteins: ___ g Carbs: ___ g Fats: ___ g	_____
DINNER	**SNACKS**	Exercise Type:
		_____
		Exercise (Minutes):
Proteins: ___ g Carbs: ___ g Fats: ___ g	Proteins: ___ g Carbs: ___ g Fats: ___ g	_____
DAILY MACROS Proteins: ___ % Carbs: ___ % Fats: ___ %		

Notes:

DAY 65 | Date: _____ Mood Check: 😃 🙂 😐 🙁 😣

BREAKFAST	LUNCH	Water:
		🥤🥤🥤🥤 🥤🥤🥤🥤
		Sleep (Hours):
Proteins: ___ g Carbs: ___ g Fats: ___ g	Proteins: ___ g Carbs: ___ g Fats: ___ g	_____
DINNER	**SNACKS**	**Exercise Type:**
		_____
		Exercise (Minutes):
Proteins: ___ g Carbs: ___ g Fats: ___ g	Proteins: ___ g Carbs: ___ g Fats: ___ g	
DAILY MACROS Proteins: ___ % Carbs: ___ % Fats: ___ %		_____

Notes:

DAY 66 | Date: _____ Mood Check: 😃 🙂 😐 🙁 😣

BREAKFAST	LUNCH	Water:
		🥤🥤🥤🥤 🥤🥤🥤🥤
		Sleep (Hours):
Proteins: ___ g Carbs: ___ g Fats: ___ g	Proteins: ___ g Carbs: ___ g Fats: ___ g	_____
DINNER	**SNACKS**	**Exercise Type:**
		_____
		Exercise (Minutes):
Proteins: ___ g Carbs: ___ g Fats: ___ g	Proteins: ___ g Carbs: ___ g Fats: ___ g	
DAILY MACROS Proteins: ___ % Carbs: ___ % Fats: ___ %		_____

Notes:

DAY 67
Date: _____ Mood Check: 😃 😊 😐 🙁 ☹️

BREAKFAST	LUNCH	Water:
		🥤🥤🥤🥤 🥤🥤🥤🥤
		Sleep (Hours):
Proteins: ___ g Carbs: ___ g Fats: ___ g	Proteins: ___ g Carbs: ___ g Fats: ___ g	_____
DINNER	SNACKS	Exercise Type: _____
		Exercise (Minutes):
Proteins: ___ g Carbs: ___ g Fats: ___ g	Proteins: ___ g Carbs: ___ g Fats: ___ g	
DAILY MACROS Proteins: ___ % Carbs: ___ % Fats: ___ %		_____

Notes:

DAY 68
Date: _____ Mood Check: 😃 😊 😐 🙁 ☹️

BREAKFAST	LUNCH	Water:
		🥤🥤🥤🥤 🥤🥤🥤🥤
		Sleep (Hours):
Proteins: ___ g Carbs: ___ g Fats: ___ g	Proteins: ___ g Carbs: ___ g Fats: ___ g	_____
DINNER	SNACKS	Exercise Type: _____
		Exercise (Minutes):
Proteins: ___ g Carbs: ___ g Fats: ___ g	Proteins: ___ g Carbs: ___ g Fats: ___ g	
DAILY MACROS Proteins: ___ % Carbs: ___ % Fats: ___ %		_____

Notes:

DAY 69 Date: _____ Mood Check: 😃 🙂 😐 🙁 ☹️

BREAKFAST	LUNCH	Water:
		🥛🥛🥛🥛🥛 🥛🥛🥛🥛🥛
		Sleep (Hours):
Proteins: ___ g Carbs: ___ g Fats: ___ g	Proteins: ___ g Carbs: ___ g Fats: ___ g	_____
DINNER	**SNACKS**	Exercise Type:
		_____
		Exercise (Minutes):
Proteins: ___ g Carbs: ___ g Fats: ___ g	Proteins: ___ g Carbs: ___ g Fats: ___ g	_____
DAILY MACROS Proteins: ___ % Carbs: ___ % Fats: ___ %		

Notes:

DAY 70 Date: _____ Mood Check: 😃 🙂 😐 🙁 ☹️

BREAKFAST	LUNCH	Water:
		🥛🥛🥛🥛🥛 🥛🥛🥛🥛🥛
		Sleep (Hours):
Proteins: ___ g Carbs: ___ g Fats: ___ g	Proteins: ___ g Carbs: ___ g Fats: ___ g	_____
DINNER	**SNACKS**	Exercise Type:
		_____
		Exercise (Minutes):
Proteins: ___ g Carbs: ___ g Fats: ___ g	Proteins: ___ g Carbs: ___ g Fats: ___ g	_____
DAILY MACROS Proteins: ___ % Carbs: ___ % Fats: ___ %		

Notes:

WEEKLY INTENTION

TARGET MACROS

What are you excited about for this week?

_____

Proteins: _____ %
Carbs: _____ %
Fats: _____ %

_____

_____

_____

What is something you'd like to work on this week? _____

_____

_____

_____

DAY 71	Date: _____	Mood Check: 😀 🙂 😐 🙁 ☹️
BREAKFAST	**LUNCH**	Water:
		Sleep (Hours):
Proteins: ___ g Carbs: ___ g Fats: ___ g	Proteins: ___ g Carbs: ___ g Fats: ___ g	_____
DINNER	**SNACKS**	Exercise Type:
		_____
		Exercise (Minutes):
Proteins: ___ g Carbs: ___ g Fats: ___ g	Proteins: ___ g Carbs: ___ g Fats: ___ g	_____
DAILY MACROS	Proteins: ___ % Carbs: ___ % Fats: ___ %	

Notes:

DAY 72 Date: _____ Mood Check: 😀 🙂 😐 🙁 ☹️

BREAKFAST	LUNCH	Water:
		🥤🥤🥤🥤 🥤🥤🥤🥤
		Sleep (Hours):
Proteins: ___ g Carbs: ___ g Fats: ___ g	Proteins: ___ g Carbs: ___ g Fats: ___ g	_____
DINNER	**SNACKS**	Exercise Type:
		_____
		Exercise (Minutes):
Proteins: ___ g Carbs: ___ g Fats: ___ g	Proteins: ___ g Carbs: ___ g Fats: ___ g	
DAILY MACROS Proteins: ___ % Carbs: ___ % Fats: ___ %		_____

Notes:

DAY 73 Date: _____ Mood Check: 😀 🙂 😐 🙁 ☹️

BREAKFAST	LUNCH	Water:
		🥤🥤🥤🥤 🥤🥤🥤🥤
		Sleep (Hours):
Proteins: ___ g Carbs: ___ g Fats: ___ g	Proteins: ___ g Carbs: ___ g Fats: ___ g	_____
DINNER	**SNACKS**	Exercise Type:
		_____
		Exercise (Minutes):
Proteins: ___ g Carbs: ___ g Fats: ___ g	Proteins: ___ g Carbs: ___ g Fats: ___ g	
DAILY MACROS Proteins: ___ % Carbs: ___ % Fats: ___ %		_____

Notes:

DAY 74 Date: _____ Mood Check: 😃 🙂 😐 🙁 ☹️

BREAKFAST	LUNCH	Water:
		🥤🥤🥤🥤 🥤🥤🥤🥤
		Sleep (Hours):
Proteins: ___ g Carbs: ___ g Fats: ___ g	Proteins: ___ g Carbs: ___ g Fats: ___ g	_____
DINNER	**SNACKS**	Exercise Type:
		_____
		Exercise (Minutes):
Proteins: ___ g Carbs: ___ g Fats: ___ g	Proteins: ___ g Carbs: ___ g Fats: ___ g	_____
DAILY MACROS Proteins: ___ % Carbs: ___ % Fats: ___ %		

Notes:

DAY 75 Date: _____ Mood Check: 😃 🙂 😐 🙁 ☹️

BREAKFAST	LUNCH	Water:
		🥤🥤🥤🥤 🥤🥤🥤🥤
		Sleep (Hours):
Proteins: ___ g Carbs: ___ g Fats: ___ g	Proteins: ___ g Carbs: ___ g Fats: ___ g	_____
DINNER	**SNACKS**	Exercise Type:
		_____
		Exercise (Minutes):
Proteins: ___ g Carbs: ___ g Fats: ___ g	Proteins: ___ g Carbs: ___ g Fats: ___ g	_____
DAILY MACROS Proteins: ___ % Carbs: ___ % Fats: ___ %		

Notes:

DAY 76 Date: _____ Mood Check: 😃 🙂 😐 🙁 😞

BREAKFAST	LUNCH	Water:
		🥛🥛🥛🥛 🥛🥛🥛🥛
		Sleep (Hours):
Proteins: ___ g Carbs: ___ g Fats: ___ g	Proteins: ___ g Carbs: ___ g Fats: ___ g	_____
DINNER	**SNACKS**	Exercise Type:
		_____
		Exercise (Minutes):
Proteins: ___ g Carbs: ___ g Fats: ___ g	Proteins: ___ g Carbs: ___ g Fats: ___ g	_____
DAILY MACROS	Proteins: ___ % Carbs: ___ % Fats: ___ %	

Notes:

DAY 77 Date: _____ Mood Check: 😃 🙂 😐 🙁 😞

BREAKFAST	LUNCH	Water:
		🥛🥛🥛🥛 🥛🥛🥛🥛
		Sleep (Hours):
Proteins: ___ g Carbs: ___ g Fats: ___ g	Proteins: ___ g Carbs: ___ g Fats: ___ g	_____
DINNER	**SNACKS**	Exercise Type:
		_____
		Exercise (Minutes):
Proteins: ___ g Carbs: ___ g Fats: ___ g	Proteins: ___ g Carbs: ___ g Fats: ___ g	_____
DAILY MACROS	Proteins: ___ % Carbs: ___ % Fats: ___ %	

Notes:

WEEKLY INTENTION

What are you excited about for this week?

Proteins: _____ %
Carbs: _____ %
Fats: _____ %

_____

_____

_____

What is something you'd like to work on this week? _____

_____

_____

_____

DAY 78	Date: _____	Mood Check: ☺ ☺ ☺ ☹ ☹
BREAKFAST	**LUNCH**	Water:
		🥛🥛🥛🥛🥛 🥛🥛🥛🥛🥛
		Sleep (Hours):
Proteins: ___ g Carbs: ___ g Fats: ___ g	Proteins: ___ g Carbs: ___ g Fats: ___ g	_____
DINNER	**SNACKS**	Exercise Type:
		_____
		Exercise (Minutes):
Proteins: ___ g Carbs: ___ g Fats: ___ g	Proteins: ___ g Carbs: ___ g Fats: ___ g	_____
DAILY MACROS Proteins: ___ % Carbs: ___ % Fats: ___ %		

Notes:

DAY 79   Date: _____   Mood Check: 😊 😊 😐 🙁 😞

BREAKFAST	LUNCH	Water:
		🥛🥛🥛🥛 🥛🥛🥛🥛
		Sleep (Hours):
Proteins: ___ g Carbs: ___ g Fats: ___ g	Proteins: ___ g Carbs: ___ g Fats: ___ g	_____
DINNER	**SNACKS**	Exercise Type:
		_____
		Exercise (Minutes):
Proteins: ___ g Carbs: ___ g Fats: ___ g	Proteins: ___ g Carbs: ___ g Fats: ___ g	_____
DAILY MACROS Proteins: ___ % Carbs: ___ % Fats: ___ %		

Notes:

DAY 80   Date: _____   Mood Check: 😊 😊 😐 🙁 😞

BREAKFAST	LUNCH	Water:
		🥛🥛🥛🥛 🥛🥛🥛🥛
		Sleep (Hours):
Proteins: ___ g Carbs: ___ g Fats: ___ g	Proteins: ___ g Carbs: ___ g Fats: ___ g	_____
DINNER	**SNACKS**	Exercise Type:
		_____
		Exercise (Minutes):
Proteins: ___ g Carbs: ___ g Fats: ___ g	Proteins: ___ g Carbs: ___ g Fats: ___ g	_____
DAILY MACROS Proteins: ___ % Carbs: ___ % Fats: ___ %		

Notes:

DAY 81   Date: _____   Mood Check: 😃 😊 😐 🙁 😣

BREAKFAST	LUNCH	Water:
		🥛🥛🥛🥛 🥛🥛🥛🥛
		Sleep (Hours):
Proteins: ___ g Carbs: ___ g Fats: ___ g	Proteins: ___ g Carbs: ___ g Fats: ___ g	
DINNER	**SNACKS**	Exercise Type:
		_____
		Exercise (Minutes):
Proteins: ___ g Carbs: ___ g Fats: ___ g	Proteins: ___ g Carbs: ___ g Fats: ___ g	
DAILY MACROS Proteins: ___ % Carbs: ___ % Fats: ___ %		

Notes:

DAY 82   Date: _____   Mood Check: 😃 😊 😐 🙁 😣

BREAKFAST	LUNCH	Water:
		🥛🥛🥛🥛 🥛🥛🥛🥛
		Sleep (Hours):
Proteins: ___ g Carbs: ___ g Fats: ___ g	Proteins: ___ g Carbs: ___ g Fats: ___ g	
DINNER	**SNACKS**	Exercise Type:
		_____
		Exercise (Minutes):
Proteins: ___ g Carbs: ___ g Fats: ___ g	Proteins: ___ g Carbs: ___ g Fats: ___ g	
DAILY MACROS Proteins: ___ % Carbs: ___ % Fats: ___ %		

Notes:

DAY 83 Date: _____ Mood Check: 😊 🙂 😐 🙁 ☹️

BREAKFAST	LUNCH	Water:
		🥛🥛🥛🥛🥛 🥛🥛🥛🥛🥛
		Sleep (Hours):
Proteins: ___ g Carbs: ___ g Fats: ___ g	Proteins: ___ g Carbs: ___ g Fats: ___ g	_____

DINNER	SNACKS	Exercise Type:
		_____
		Exercise (Minutes):
Proteins: ___ g Carbs: ___ g Fats: ___ g	Proteins: ___ g Carbs: ___ g Fats: ___ g	

DAILY MACROS	Proteins: ___ % Carbs: ___ % Fats: ___ %	_____

Notes:

DAY 84 Date: _____ Mood Check: 😊 🙂 😐 🙁 ☹️

BREAKFAST	LUNCH	Water:
		🥛🥛🥛🥛🥛 🥛🥛🥛🥛🥛
		Sleep (Hours):
Proteins: ___ g Carbs: ___ g Fats: ___ g	Proteins: ___ g Carbs: ___ g Fats: ___ g	_____

DINNER	SNACKS	Exercise Type:
		_____
		Exercise (Minutes):
Proteins: ___ g Carbs: ___ g Fats: ___ g	Proteins: ___ g Carbs: ___ g Fats: ___ g	

DAILY MACROS	Proteins: ___ % Carbs: ___ % Fats: ___ %	_____

Notes:

FOUR-WEEK CHECK-IN

Date: _____

MEASUREMENT	CURRENT	MONTH CHANGE
WEIGHT (LB)		
UPPER ARMS (IN)		
CHEST (IN)		
WAIST (IN)		
HIPS (IN)		
THIGHS (IN)		
CALVES (IN)		

CONGRATULATIONS ON MAKING IT THIS FAR!

What are you most proud of accomplishing in the past four weeks?

_____

_____

_____

_____

What was your biggest challenge over the past four weeks?

_____

_____

_____

_____

_____

What are some goals you would like to work toward for the next four weeks?

_____

_____

_____

_____

Reflect on your mood over the past month. Did you notice differences related to your eating habits?

_____

_____

_____

_____

_____

WEEKLY INTENTION

What are you excited about for this week?

Proteins: _____ %
Carbs: _____ %
Fats: _____ %

_____

_____

_____

What is something you'd like to work on this week? _____

_____

_____

DAY 85	Date: _____	Mood Check: 😃 🙂 😐 🙁 😞
BREAKFAST	**LUNCH**	Water:
		Sleep (Hours):
Proteins: ___ g Carbs: ___ g Fats: ___ g	Proteins: ___ g Carbs: ___ g Fats: ___ g	_____
DINNER	**SNACKS**	Exercise Type: _____
		Exercise (Minutes):
Proteins: ___ g Carbs: ___ g Fats: ___ g	Proteins: ___ g Carbs: ___ g Fats: ___ g	_____
DAILY MACROS Proteins: ___ % Carbs: ___ % Fats: ___ %		

Notes:

DAY 86   Date: _____   Mood Check: 😄 🙂 😐 🙁 😟

BREAKFAST	LUNCH	Water:
		🥛🥛🥛🥛 🥛🥛🥛🥛
		Sleep (Hours):
Proteins: ___ g Carbs: ___ g Fats: ___ g	Proteins: ___ g Carbs: ___ g Fats: ___ g	_____
DINNER	SNACKS	Exercise Type:
		_____
		Exercise (Minutes):
Proteins: ___ g Carbs: ___ g Fats: ___ g	Proteins: ___ g Carbs: ___ g Fats: ___ g	_____
DAILY MACROS Proteins: ___ % Carbs: ___ % Fats: ___ %		

Notes:

DAY 87   Date: _____   Mood Check: 😄 🙂 😐 🙁 😟

BREAKFAST	LUNCH	Water:
		🥛🥛🥛🥛 🥛🥛🥛🥛
		Sleep (Hours):
Proteins: ___ g Carbs: ___ g Fats: ___ g	Proteins: ___ g Carbs: ___ g Fats: ___ g	_____
DINNER	SNACKS	Exercise Type:
		_____
		Exercise (Minutes):
Proteins: ___ g Carbs: ___ g Fats: ___ g	Proteins: ___ g Carbs: ___ g Fats: ___ g	_____
DAILY MACROS Proteins: ___ % Carbs: ___ % Fats: ___ %		

Notes:

DAY 88 Date: _____ Mood Check: 😃 😊 😐 🙁 ☹️

BREAKFAST	LUNCH	Water:
		🥛🥛🥛🥛 🥛🥛🥛🥛
		Sleep (Hours):
Proteins: ___ g Carbs: ___ g Fats: ___ g	Proteins: ___ g Carbs: ___ g Fats: ___ g	_____
DINNER	SNACKS	Exercise Type:
		_____
		Exercise (Minutes):
Proteins: ___ g Carbs: ___ g Fats: ___ g	Proteins: ___ g Carbs: ___ g Fats: ___ g	
DAILY MACROS Proteins: ___ % Carbs: ___ % Fats: ___ %		_____

Notes:

DAY 89 Date: _____ Mood Check: 😃 😊 😐 🙁 ☹️

BREAKFAST	LUNCH	Water:
		🥛🥛🥛🥛 🥛🥛🥛🥛
		Sleep (Hours):
Proteins: ___ g Carbs: ___ g Fats: ___ g	Proteins: ___ g Carbs: ___ g Fats: ___ g	_____
DINNER	SNACKS	Exercise Type:
		_____
		Exercise (Minutes):
Proteins: ___ g Carbs: ___ g Fats: ___ g	Proteins: ___ g Carbs: ___ g Fats: ___ g	
DAILY MACROS Proteins: ___ % Carbs: ___ % Fats: ___ %		_____

Notes:

DAY 90   Date: _____   Mood Check: 😃 🙂 😐 🙁 😫

BREAKFAST	LUNCH	Water:
		🥛🥛🥛🥛 🥛🥛🥛🥛
		Sleep (Hours):
Proteins: ___ g Carbs: ___ g Fats: ___ g	Proteins: ___ g Carbs: ___ g Fats: ___ g	_____
DINNER	**SNACKS**	Exercise Type:
		_____
		Exercise (Minutes):
Proteins: ___ g Carbs: ___ g Fats: ___ g	Proteins: ___ g Carbs: ___ g Fats: ___ g	
DAILY MACROS Proteins: ___ % Carbs: ___ % Fats: ___ %		

Notes:

DAY 91   Date: _____   Mood Check: 😃 🙂 😐 🙁 😫

BREAKFAST	LUNCH	Water:
		🥛🥛🥛🥛 🥛🥛🥛🥛
		Sleep (Hours):
Proteins: ___ g Carbs: ___ g Fats: ___ g	Proteins: ___ g Carbs: ___ g Fats: ___ g	_____
DINNER	**SNACKS**	Exercise Type:
		_____
		Exercise (Minutes):
Proteins: ___ g Carbs: ___ g Fats: ___ g	Proteins: ___ g Carbs: ___ g Fats: ___ g	
DAILY MACROS Proteins: ___ % Carbs: ___ % Fats: ___ %		

Notes:

WEEKLY INTENTION

What are you excited about for this week?

Proteins: _____ %
Carbs: _____ %
Fats: _____ %

_____

_____

_____

What is something you'd like to work on this week? _____

_____

_____

DAY 92	Date: _____	Mood Check: 😃 🙂 😐 🙁 ☹️

BREAKFAST	LUNCH	Water:
		🥛🥛🥛🥛 🥛🥛🥛🥛
		Sleep (Hours):
Proteins: ___ g Carbs: ___ g Fats: ___ g	Proteins: ___ g Carbs: ___ g Fats: ___ g	_____
DINNER	SNACKS	Exercise Type:
		_____
		Exercise (Minutes):
Proteins: ___ g Carbs: ___ g Fats: ___ g	Proteins: ___ g Carbs: ___ g Fats: ___ g	_____
DAILY MACROS	Proteins: ___ % Carbs: ___ % Fats: ___ %	

Notes:

DAY 93 | Date: _____ Mood Check: 😀 🙂 😐 🙁 😢

BREAKFAST	LUNCH	Water:
		🥛🥛🥛🥛🥛🥛🥛🥛🥛🥛
		Sleep (Hours):
Proteins: ___ g Carbs: ___ g Fats: ___ g	Proteins: ___ g Carbs: ___ g Fats: ___ g	_____
DINNER	SNACKS	Exercise Type:
		_____
		Exercise (Minutes):
Proteins: ___ g Carbs: ___ g Fats: ___ g	Proteins: ___ g Carbs: ___ g Fats: ___ g	_____
DAILY MACROS Proteins: ___ % Carbs: ___ % Fats: ___ %		

Notes:

DAY 94 | Date: _____ Mood Check: 😀 🙂 😐 🙁 😢

BREAKFAST	LUNCH	Water:
		🥛🥛🥛🥛🥛🥛🥛🥛🥛🥛
		Sleep (Hours):
Proteins: ___ g Carbs: ___ g Fats: ___ g	Proteins: ___ g Carbs: ___ g Fats: ___ g	_____
DINNER	SNACKS	Exercise Type:
		_____
		Exercise (Minutes):
Proteins: ___ g Carbs: ___ g Fats: ___ g	Proteins: ___ g Carbs: ___ g Fats: ___ g	_____
DAILY MACROS Proteins: ___ % Carbs: ___ % Fats: ___ %		

Notes:

DAY 95   Date: _____   Mood Check: 😃 🙂 😐 🙁 ☹️

BREAKFAST

LUNCH

Proteins: ___ g Carbs: ___ g Fats: ___ g

Proteins: ___ g Carbs: ___ g Fats: ___ g

DINNER

SNACKS

Proteins: ___ g Carbs: ___ g Fats: ___ g

Proteins: ___ g Carbs: ___ g Fats: ___ g

DAILY MACROS   Proteins: ___ %   Carbs: ___ %   Fats: ___ %

Water:

Sleep (Hours):
_____

Exercise
Type:
_____

Exercise
(Minutes):
_____

Notes:

DAY 96   Date: _____   Mood Check: 😃 🙂 😐 🙁 ☹️

BREAKFAST

LUNCH

Proteins: ___ g Carbs: ___ g Fats: ___ g

Proteins: ___ g Carbs: ___ g Fats: ___ g

DINNER

SNACKS

Proteins: ___ g Carbs: ___ g Fats: ___ g

Proteins: ___ g Carbs: ___ g Fats: ___ g

DAILY MACROS   Proteins: ___ %   Carbs: ___ %   Fats: ___ %

Water:

Sleep (Hours):
_____

Exercise
Type:
_____

Exercise
(Minutes):
_____

Notes:

DAY 97 Date: _____ Mood Check: 😃 🙂 😐 🙁 😞

BREAKFAST	LUNCH	Water:
		🥛🥛🥛🥛🥛🥛🥛🥛🥛🥛
		Sleep (Hours):
Proteins: ___ g Carbs: ___ g Fats: ___ g	Proteins: ___ g Carbs: ___ g Fats: ___ g	
DINNER	SNACKS	Exercise Type:
		_____
		Exercise (Minutes):
Proteins: ___ g Carbs: ___ g Fats: ___ g	Proteins: ___ g Carbs: ___ g Fats: ___ g	
DAILY MACROS Proteins: ___ % Carbs: ___ % Fats: ___ %		

Notes:

DAY 98 Date: _____ Mood Check: 😃 🙂 😐 🙁 😞

BREAKFAST	LUNCH	Water:
		🥛🥛🥛🥛🥛🥛🥛🥛🥛🥛
		Sleep (Hours):
Proteins: ___ g Carbs: ___ g Fats: ___ g	Proteins: ___ g Carbs: ___ g Fats: ___ g	
DINNER	SNACKS	Exercise Type:
		_____
		Exercise (Minutes):
Proteins: ___ g Carbs: ___ g Fats: ___ g	Proteins: ___ g Carbs: ___ g Fats: ___ g	
DAILY MACROS Proteins: ___ % Carbs: ___ % Fats: ___ %		

Notes:

WEEKLY INTENTION

What are you excited about for this week?

Proteins: _____ %
Carbs: _____ %
Fats: _____ %

_____

_____

_____

What is something you'd like to work on this week? _____

_____

_____

_____

DAY 99	Date: _____	Mood Check: ☺ ☺ ☺ ☹ ☹
BREAKFAST	**LUNCH**	Water:
		🥛🥛🥛🥛🥛
		🥛🥛🥛🥛🥛
		Sleep (Hours):
Proteins: ___ g Carbs: ___ g Fats: ___ g	Proteins: ___ g Carbs: ___ g Fats: ___ g	_____
DINNER	**SNACKS**	Exercise Type:
		_____
		Exercise (Minutes):
Proteins: ___ g Carbs: ___ g Fats: ___ g	Proteins: ___ g Carbs: ___ g Fats: ___ g	
DAILY MACROS Proteins: ___ % Carbs: ___ % Fats: ___ %		_____

Notes:

DAY 100

Date: _____ Mood Check: 😃 🙂 😐 🙁 ☹️

BREAKFAST

Proteins: ___ g Carbs: ___ g Fats: ___ g

LUNCH

Proteins: ___ g Carbs: ___ g Fats: ___ g

DINNER

Proteins: ___ g Carbs: ___ g Fats: ___ g

SNACKS

Proteins: ___ g Carbs: ___ g Fats: ___ g

DAILY MACROS Proteins: ___ % Carbs: ___ % Fats: ___ %

Water:

Sleep (Hours):

_____

Exercise Type:

_____

Exercise (Minutes):

_____

Notes:

DAY 101

Date: _____ Mood Check: 😃 🙂 😐 🙁 ☹️

BREAKFAST

Proteins: ___ g Carbs: ___ g Fats: ___ g

LUNCH

Proteins: ___ g Carbs: ___ g Fats: ___ g

DINNER

Proteins: ___ g Carbs: ___ g Fats: ___ g

SNACKS

Proteins: ___ g Carbs: ___ g Fats: ___ g

DAILY MACROS Proteins: ___ % Carbs: ___ % Fats: ___ %

Water:

Sleep (Hours):

_____

Exercise Type:

_____

Exercise (Minutes):

_____

Notes:

DAY 102

Date: _____ Mood Check: 😃 😊 😐 🙁 😞

BREAKFAST	LUNCH	Water:
		🥛🥛🥛🥛 🥛🥛🥛🥛
		Sleep (Hours):
Proteins: ___ g Carbs: ___ g Fats: ___ g	Proteins: ___ g Carbs: ___ g Fats: ___ g	_____
DINNER	**SNACKS**	Exercise Type:
		_____
		Exercise (Minutes):
Proteins: ___ g Carbs: ___ g Fats: ___ g	Proteins: ___ g Carbs: ___ g Fats: ___ g	_____
DAILY MACROS Proteins: ___ % Carbs: ___ % Fats: ___ %		

Notes:

DAY 103

Date: _____ Mood Check: 😃 😊 😐 🙁 😞

BREAKFAST	LUNCH	Water:
		🥛🥛🥛🥛 🥛🥛🥛🥛
		Sleep (Hours):
Proteins: ___ g Carbs: ___ g Fats: ___ g	Proteins: ___ g Carbs: ___ g Fats: ___ g	_____
DINNER	**SNACKS**	Exercise Type:
		_____
		Exercise (Minutes):
Proteins: ___ g Carbs: ___ g Fats: ___ g	Proteins: ___ g Carbs: ___ g Fats: ___ g	_____
DAILY MACROS Proteins: ___ % Carbs: ___ % Fats: ___ %		

Notes:

DAY 104

Date: _____   Mood Check: 😊 🙂 😐 🙁 ☹️

BREAKFAST	LUNCH	Water:
		🥛🥛🥛🥛 🥛🥛🥛🥛
		Sleep (Hours):
Proteins: ___ g Carbs: ___ g Fats: ___ g	Proteins: ___ g Carbs: ___ g Fats: ___ g	_____
DINNER	**SNACKS**	Exercise Type:
		_____
		Exercise (Minutes):
Proteins: ___ g Carbs: ___ g Fats: ___ g	Proteins: ___ g Carbs: ___ g Fats: ___ g	
DAILY MACROS Proteins: ___ % Carbs: ___ % Fats: ___ %		_____

Notes:

DAY 105

Date: _____   Mood Check: 😊 🙂 😐 🙁 ☹️

BREAKFAST	LUNCH	Water:
		🥛🥛🥛🥛 🥛🥛🥛🥛
		Sleep (Hours):
Proteins: ___ g Carbs: ___ g Fats: ___ g	Proteins: ___ g Carbs: ___ g Fats: ___ g	_____
DINNER	**SNACKS**	Exercise Type:
		_____
		Exercise (Minutes):
Proteins: ___ g Carbs: ___ g Fats: ___ g	Proteins: ___ g Carbs: ___ g Fats: ___ g	
DAILY MACROS Proteins: ___ % Carbs: ___ % Fats: ___ %		_____

Notes:

WEEKLY INTENTION

What are you excited about for this week?

Proteins: _____ %
Carbs: _____ %
Fats: _____ %

_____

_____

_____

What is something you'd like to work on this week? _____

_____

_____

_____

DAY 106	Date: _____	Mood Check: 😀 🙂 😐 🙁 😣

BREAKFAST	LUNCH	Water:
		🥛🥛🥛🥛🥛 🥛🥛🥛🥛🥛
		Sleep (Hours):
Proteins: ___ g Carbs: ___ g Fats: ___ g	Proteins: ___ g Carbs: ___ g Fats: ___ g	_____
DINNER	SNACKS	Exercise Type:
		_____
		Exercise (Minutes):
Proteins: ___ g Carbs: ___ g Fats: ___ g	Proteins: ___ g Carbs: ___ g Fats: ___ g	
DAILY MACROS	Proteins: ___ % Carbs: ___ % Fats: ___ %	_____

Notes:

DAY 107 Date: _____ Mood Check: 😀 🙂 😐 🙁 ☹️

BREAKFAST	LUNCH	Water:
		🥛 🥛 🥛 🥛 🥛
		🥛 🥛 🥛 🥛 🥛
		Sleep (Hours):
Proteins: ___ g Carbs: ___ g Fats: ___ g	Proteins: ___ g Carbs: ___ g Fats: ___ g	_____
DINNER	SNACKS	Exercise Type:
		_____
		Exercise (Minutes):
Proteins: ___ g Carbs: ___ g Fats: ___ g	Proteins: ___ g Carbs: ___ g Fats: ___ g	_____
DAILY MACROS Proteins: ___ % Carbs: ___ % Fats: ___ %		

Notes:

DAY 108 Date: _____ Mood Check: 😀 🙂 😐 🙁 ☹️

BREAKFAST	LUNCH	Water:
		🥛 🥛 🥛 🥛 🥛
		🥛 🥛 🥛 🥛 🥛
		Sleep (Hours):
Proteins: ___ g Carbs: ___ g Fats: ___ g	Proteins: ___ g Carbs: ___ g Fats: ___ g	_____
DINNER	SNACKS	Exercise Type:
		_____
		Exercise (Minutes):
Proteins: ___ g Carbs: ___ g Fats: ___ g	Proteins: ___ g Carbs: ___ g Fats: ___ g	_____
DAILY MACROS Proteins: ___ % Carbs: ___ % Fats: ___ %		

Notes:

DAY 109 Date: _____ Mood Check: 😃 🙂 😐 🙁 ☹️

BREAKFAST

LUNCH

Water:

Sleep (Hours):

_____

Proteins: ___ g Carbs: ___ g Fats: ___ g

Proteins: ___ g Carbs: ___ g Fats: ___ g

DINNER

SNACKS

Exercise Type:

_____

Exercise (Minutes):

Proteins: ___ g Carbs: ___ g Fats: ___ g

Proteins: ___ g Carbs: ___ g Fats: ___ g

DAILY MACROS   Proteins: ___ %   Carbs: ___ %   Fats: ___ %

_____

Notes:

DAY 110 Date: _____ Mood Check: 😃 🙂 😐 🙁 ☹️

BREAKFAST

LUNCH

Water:

Sleep (Hours):

_____

Proteins: ___ g Carbs: ___ g Fats: ___ g

Proteins: ___ g Carbs: ___ g Fats: ___ g

DINNER

SNACKS

Exercise Type:

_____

Exercise (Minutes):

Proteins: ___ g Carbs: ___ g Fats: ___ g

Proteins: ___ g Carbs: ___ g Fats: ___ g

DAILY MACROS   Proteins: ___ %   Carbs: ___ %   Fats: ___ %

_____

Notes:

DAY 111 Date: _____ Mood Check: 😀 🙂 😐 🙁 😣

BREAKFAST	LUNCH	Water:
		🥛🥛🥛🥛 🥛🥛🥛🥛
		Sleep (Hours):
Proteins: ___ g Carbs: ___ g Fats: ___ g	Proteins: ___ g Carbs: ___ g Fats: ___ g	_____
DINNER	**SNACKS**	Exercise Type:
		_____
		Exercise (Minutes):
Proteins: ___ g Carbs: ___ g Fats: ___ g	Proteins: ___ g Carbs: ___ g Fats: ___ g	
DAILY MACROS Proteins: ___ % Carbs: ___ % Fats: ___ %		_____

Notes:

DAY 112 Date: _____ Mood Check: 😀 🙂 😐 🙁 😣

BREAKFAST	LUNCH	Water:
		🥛🥛🥛🥛 🥛🥛🥛🥛
		Sleep (Hours):
Proteins: ___ g Carbs: ___ g Fats: ___ g	Proteins: ___ g Carbs: ___ g Fats: ___ g	_____
DINNER	**SNACKS**	Exercise Type:
		_____
		Exercise (Minutes):
Proteins: ___ g Carbs: ___ g Fats: ___ g	Proteins: ___ g Carbs: ___ g Fats: ___ g	
DAILY MACROS Proteins: ___ % Carbs: ___ % Fats: ___ %		_____

Notes:

FOUR-WEEK CHECK-IN

Date: _____

MEASUREMENT	CURRENT	MONTH CHANGE
WEIGHT (LB)		
UPPER ARMS (IN)		
CHEST (IN)		
WAIST (IN)		
HIPS (IN)		
THIGHS (IN)		
CALVES (IN)		

CONGRATULATIONS ON MAKING IT THIS FAR!

What are you most proud of accomplishing in the past four weeks?

_____

_____

_____

_____

What was your biggest challenge over the past four weeks?

_____

_____

_____

_____

_____

What are some goals you would like to work toward for the next four weeks?

_____

_____

_____

_____

Reflect on your mood over the past month. Did you notice differences related to your eating habits?

_____

_____

_____

_____

_____

WEEKLY INTENTION

What are you excited about for this week?

Proteins: _____ %
Carbs: _____ %
Fats: _____ %

_____

_____

_____

_____

What is something you'd like to work on this week? _____

_____

_____

_____

DAY 113	Date: _____	Mood Check: 😃 🙂 😐 🙁 😞

BREAKFAST

LUNCH

Water:

Sleep (Hours):

Proteins: ___ g Carbs: ___ g Fats: ___ g

Proteins: ___ g Carbs: ___ g Fats: ___ g

_____

DINNER

SNACKS

Exercise Type:

_____

Exercise (Minutes):

Proteins: ___ g Carbs: ___ g Fats: ___ g

Proteins: ___ g Carbs: ___ g Fats: ___ g

DAILY MACROS Proteins: ___ % Carbs: ___ % Fats: ___ %

_____

Notes:

DAY 114   Date: _____   Mood Check: 😃 😊 😐 🙁 😞

BREAKFAST	LUNCH	Water:
		🥛🥛🥛🥛 🥛🥛🥛🥛
		Sleep (Hours):
Proteins: ___ g Carbs: ___ g Fats: ___ g	Proteins: ___ g Carbs: ___ g Fats: ___ g	_____
DINNER	SNACKS	Exercise Type:
		_____
		Exercise (Minutes):
Proteins: ___ g Carbs: ___ g Fats: ___ g	Proteins: ___ g Carbs: ___ g Fats: ___ g	_____
DAILY MACROS Proteins: ___ % Carbs: ___ % Fats: ___ %		

Notes:

DAY 115   Date: _____   Mood Check: 😃 😊 😐 🙁 😞

BREAKFAST	LUNCH	Water:
		🥛🥛🥛🥛 🥛🥛🥛🥛
		Sleep (Hours):
Proteins: ___ g Carbs: ___ g Fats: ___ g	Proteins: ___ g Carbs: ___ g Fats: ___ g	_____
DINNER	SNACKS	Exercise Type:
		_____
		Exercise (Minutes):
Proteins: ___ g Carbs: ___ g Fats: ___ g	Proteins: ___ g Carbs: ___ g Fats: ___ g	_____
DAILY MACROS Proteins: ___ % Carbs: ___ % Fats: ___ %		

Notes:

DAY 116

Date: _____   Mood Check: 😃 😊 😐 🙁 ☹️

BREAKFAST

LUNCH

Water:

Sleep (Hours):

_____

Proteins: ___ g Carbs: ___ g Fats: ___ g

Proteins: ___ g Carbs: ___ g Fats: ___ g

DINNER

SNACKS

Exercise Type:

_____

Exercise (Minutes):

Proteins: ___ g Carbs: ___ g Fats: ___ g

Proteins: ___ g Carbs: ___ g Fats: ___ g

DAILY MACROS   Proteins: ___ % Carbs: ___ % Fats: ___ %

_____

Notes:

DAY 117

Date: _____   Mood Check: 😃 😊 😐 🙁 ☹️

BREAKFAST

LUNCH

Water:

Sleep (Hours):

_____

Proteins: ___ g Carbs: ___ g Fats: ___ g

Proteins: ___ g Carbs: ___ g Fats: ___ g

DINNER

SNACKS

Exercise Type:

_____

Exercise (Minutes):

Proteins: ___ g Carbs: ___ g Fats: ___ g

Proteins: ___ g Carbs: ___ g Fats: ___ g

DAILY MACROS   Proteins: ___ % Carbs: ___ % Fats: ___ %

_____

Notes:

DAY 118 Date: _____ Mood Check: 😃 🙂 😐 🙁 😣

BREAKFAST	LUNCH	Water:
		🥤🥤🥤🥤 🥤🥤🥤🥤
		Sleep (Hours):
Proteins: ___ g Carbs: ___ g Fats: ___ g	Proteins: ___ g Carbs: ___ g Fats: ___ g	_____
DINNER	**SNACKS**	Exercise Type:
		_____
		Exercise (Minutes):
Proteins: ___ g Carbs: ___ g Fats: ___ g	Proteins: ___ g Carbs: ___ g Fats: ___ g	
DAILY MACROS Proteins: ___ % Carbs: ___ % Fats: ___ %		_____

Notes:

DAY 119 Date: _____ Mood Check: 😃 🙂 😐 🙁 😣

BREAKFAST	LUNCH	Water:
		🥤🥤🥤🥤 🥤🥤🥤🥤
		Sleep (Hours):
Proteins: ___ g Carbs: ___ g Fats: ___ g	Proteins: ___ g Carbs: ___ g Fats: ___ g	_____
DINNER	**SNACKS**	Exercise Type:
		_____
		Exercise (Minutes):
Proteins: ___ g Carbs: ___ g Fats: ___ g	Proteins: ___ g Carbs: ___ g Fats: ___ g	
DAILY MACROS Proteins: ___ % Carbs: ___ % Fats: ___ %		_____

Notes:

WEEK 18

WEEKLY INTENTION

TARGET MACROS

What are you excited about for this week?

Proteins: _____ %
Carbs: _____ %
Fats: _____ %

_____

_____

_____

What is something you'd like to work on this week? _____

_____

_____

_____

DAY 120	Date: _____	Mood Check: 😀 🙂 😐 🙁 ☹️
BREAKFAST	**LUNCH**	Water: 🥛🥛🥛🥛 🥛🥛🥛🥛
		Sleep (Hours):
Proteins: ___ g Carbs: ___ g Fats: ___ g	Proteins: ___ g Carbs: ___ g Fats: ___ g	_____
DINNER	**SNACKS**	Exercise Type: _____
		Exercise (Minutes):
Proteins: ___ g Carbs: ___ g Fats: ___ g	Proteins: ___ g Carbs: ___ g Fats: ___ g	_____
DAILY MACROS	Proteins: ___ % Carbs: ___ % Fats: ___ %	

Notes:

DAY 121 Date: _____ Mood Check: 😃 😊 😐 😣 😞

BREAKFAST	LUNCH	Water:
		🥛🥛🥛🥛🥛🥛🥛🥛
		Sleep (Hours):
Proteins: ___ g Carbs: ___ g Fats: ___ g	Proteins: ___ g Carbs: ___ g Fats: ___ g	_____
DINNER	**SNACKS**	Exercise Type:
		_____
		Exercise (Minutes):
Proteins: ___ g Carbs: ___ g Fats: ___ g	Proteins: ___ g Carbs: ___ g Fats: ___ g	_____
DAILY MACROS Proteins: ___ % Carbs: ___ % Fats: ___ %		

Notes:

DAY 122 Date: _____ Mood Check: 😃 😊 😐 😣 😞

BREAKFAST	LUNCH	Water:
		🥛🥛🥛🥛🥛🥛🥛🥛
		Sleep (Hours):
Proteins: ___ g Carbs: ___ g Fats: ___ g	Proteins: ___ g Carbs: ___ g Fats: ___ g	_____
DINNER	**SNACKS**	Exercise Type:
		_____
		Exercise (Minutes):
Proteins: ___ g Carbs: ___ g Fats: ___ g	Proteins: ___ g Carbs: ___ g Fats: ___ g	_____
DAILY MACROS Proteins: ___ % Carbs: ___ % Fats: ___ %		

Notes:

DAY 123

Date: _____ Mood Check: 😀 🙂 😐 🙁 😫

BREAKFAST	LUNCH	Water:
		🥛🥛🥛🥛 🥛🥛🥛🥛
		Sleep (Hours):
Proteins: ___ g Carbs: ___ g Fats: ___ g	Proteins: ___ g Carbs: ___ g Fats: ___ g	_____
DINNER	SNACKS	Exercise Type:
		_____
		Exercise (Minutes):
Proteins: ___ g Carbs: ___ g Fats: ___ g	Proteins: ___ g Carbs: ___ g Fats: ___ g	_____
DAILY MACROS	Proteins: ___ % Carbs: ___ % Fats: ___ %	

Notes:

DAY 124

Date: _____ Mood Check: 😀 🙂 😐 🙁 😫

BREAKFAST	LUNCH	Water:
		🥛🥛🥛🥛 🥛🥛🥛🥛
		Sleep (Hours):
Proteins: ___ g Carbs: ___ g Fats: ___ g	Proteins: ___ g Carbs: ___ g Fats: ___ g	_____
DINNER	SNACKS	Exercise Type:
		_____
		Exercise (Minutes):
Proteins: ___ g Carbs: ___ g Fats: ___ g	Proteins: ___ g Carbs: ___ g Fats: ___ g	_____
DAILY MACROS	Proteins: ___ % Carbs: ___ % Fats: ___ %	

Notes:

DAY 125   Date: _____   Mood Check: 😀 🙂 😐 🙁 😫

BREAKFAST	LUNCH	Water:
		🥛🥛🥛🥛 🥛🥛🥛🥛
		Sleep (Hours):
Proteins: ___ g Carbs: ___ g Fats: ___ g	Proteins: ___ g Carbs: ___ g Fats: ___ g	_____
DINNER	**SNACKS**	Exercise Type:
		_____
		Exercise (Minutes):
Proteins: ___ g Carbs: ___ g Fats: ___ g	Proteins: ___ g Carbs: ___ g Fats: ___ g	_____
DAILY MACROS Proteins: ___ % Carbs: ___ % Fats: ___ %		

Notes:

DAY 126   Date: _____   Mood Check: 😀 🙂 😐 🙁 😫

BREAKFAST	LUNCH	Water:
		🥛🥛🥛🥛 🥛🥛🥛🥛
		Sleep (Hours):
Proteins: ___ g Carbs: ___ g Fats: ___ g	Proteins: ___ g Carbs: ___ g Fats: ___ g	_____
DINNER	**SNACKS**	Exercise Type:
		_____
		Exercise (Minutes):
Proteins: ___ g Carbs: ___ g Fats: ___ g	Proteins: ___ g Carbs: ___ g Fats: ___ g	_____
DAILY MACROS Proteins: ___ % Carbs: ___ % Fats: ___ %		

Notes:

WEEK 19

WEEKLY INTENTION

TARGET MACROS

What are you excited about for this week?

Proteins: _____ %
Carbs: _____ %
Fats: _____ %

_____

_____

_____

What is something you'd like to work on this week? _____

_____

_____

_____

DAY 127	Date: _____	Mood Check: 😀 🙂 😐 🙁 ☹️
BREAKFAST	**LUNCH**	Water:
		🥛🥛🥛🥛🥛 🥛🥛🥛🥛🥛
		Sleep (Hours):
Proteins: ___g Carbs: ___g Fats: ___g	Proteins: ___g Carbs: ___g Fats: ___g	_____
DINNER	**SNACKS**	Exercise Type: _____
		Exercise (Minutes):
Proteins: ___g Carbs: ___g Fats: ___g	Proteins: ___g Carbs: ___g Fats: ___g	_____
DAILY MACROS	Proteins: ___% Carbs: ___% Fats: ___%	

Notes:

DAY 128   Date: _____   Mood Check: 😃 🙂 😐 🙁 😣

BREAKFAST	LUNCH	Water:
		🥛🥛🥛🥛 🥛🥛🥛🥛
		Sleep (Hours):
Proteins: ___ g Carbs: ___ g Fats: ___ g	Proteins: ___ g Carbs: ___ g Fats: ___ g	_____
DINNER	**SNACKS**	Exercise Type:
		_____
		Exercise (Minutes):
Proteins: ___ g Carbs: ___ g Fats: ___ g	Proteins: ___ g Carbs: ___ g Fats: ___ g	_____
DAILY MACROS Proteins: ___ % Carbs: ___ % Fats: ___ %		

Notes:

DAY 129   Date: _____   Mood Check: 😃 🙂 😐 🙁 😣

BREAKFAST	LUNCH	Water:
		🥛🥛🥛🥛 🥛🥛🥛🥛
		Sleep (Hours):
Proteins: ___ g Carbs: ___ g Fats: ___ g	Proteins: ___ g Carbs: ___ g Fats: ___ g	_____
DINNER	**SNACKS**	Exercise Type:
		_____
		Exercise (Minutes):
Proteins: ___ g Carbs: ___ g Fats: ___ g	Proteins: ___ g Carbs: ___ g Fats: ___ g	_____
DAILY MACROS Proteins: ___ % Carbs: ___ % Fats: ___ %		

Notes:

DAY 130

Date: _____   Mood Check: 😀 🙂 😐 🙁 😞

BREAKFAST	LUNCH	Water:
		🥛🥛🥛🥛 🥛🥛🥛🥛
		Sleep (Hours):
Proteins: ___ g Carbs: ___ g Fats: ___ g	Proteins: ___ g Carbs: ___ g Fats: ___ g	_____
DINNER	**SNACKS**	Exercise Type:
		_____
		Exercise (Minutes):
Proteins: ___ g Carbs: ___ g Fats: ___ g	Proteins: ___ g Carbs: ___ g Fats: ___ g	_____
DAILY MACROS Proteins: ___ % Carbs: ___ % Fats: ___ %		

Notes:

DAY 131

Date: _____   Mood Check: 😀 🙂 😐 🙁 😞

BREAKFAST	LUNCH	Water:
		🥛🥛🥛🥛 🥛🥛🥛🥛
		Sleep (Hours):
Proteins: ___ g Carbs: ___ g Fats: ___ g	Proteins: ___ g Carbs: ___ g Fats: ___ g	_____
DINNER	**SNACKS**	Exercise Type:
		_____
		Exercise (Minutes):
Proteins: ___ g Carbs: ___ g Fats: ___ g	Proteins: ___ g Carbs: ___ g Fats: ___ g	_____
DAILY MACROS Proteins: ___ % Carbs: ___ % Fats: ___ %		

Notes:

DAY 132   Date: _____   Mood Check: 😀 🙂 😐 🙁 ☹️

BREAKFAST	LUNCH	Water:
		🥛🥛🥛🥛🥛 🥛🥛🥛🥛🥛
		Sleep (Hours):
Proteins: ___ g Carbs: ___ g Fats: ___ g	Proteins: ___ g Carbs: ___ g Fats: ___ g	_____
DINNER	**SNACKS**	Exercise Type:
		_____
		Exercise (Minutes):
Proteins: ___ g Carbs: ___ g Fats: ___ g	Proteins: ___ g Carbs: ___ g Fats: ___ g	
DAILY MACROS Proteins: ___ % Carbs: ___ % Fats: ___ %		_____

Notes:

DAY 133   Date: _____   Mood Check: 😀 🙂 😐 🙁 ☹️

BREAKFAST	LUNCH	Water:
		🥛🥛🥛🥛🥛 🥛🥛🥛🥛🥛
		Sleep (Hours):
Proteins: ___ g Carbs: ___ g Fats: ___ g	Proteins: ___ g Carbs: ___ g Fats: ___ g	_____
DINNER	**SNACKS**	Exercise Type:
		_____
		Exercise (Minutes):
Proteins: ___ g Carbs: ___ g Fats: ___ g	Proteins: ___ g Carbs: ___ g Fats: ___ g	
DAILY MACROS Proteins: ___ % Carbs: ___ % Fats: ___ %		_____

Notes:

WEEKLY INTENTION

What are you excited about for this week?

Proteins: _____ %
Carbs: _____ %
Fats: _____ %

_____

_____

_____

What is something you'd like to work on this week? _____

_____

_____

_____

DAY 134	Date: _____	Mood Check: ☺ ☺ 😐 ☹ ☹
BREAKFAST	**LUNCH**	Water:
		Sleep (Hours):
Proteins: ___ g Carbs: ___ g Fats: ___ g	Proteins: ___ g Carbs: ___ g Fats: ___ g	
DINNER	**SNACKS**	Exercise Type:
		Exercise (Minutes):
Proteins: ___ g Carbs: ___ g Fats: ___ g	Proteins: ___ g Carbs: ___ g Fats: ___ g	
DAILY MACROS Proteins: ___ % Carbs: ___ % Fats: ___ %		

Notes:

DAY 135 Date: _____ Mood Check: 😀 🙂 😐 🙁 ☹️

BREAKFAST	LUNCH	Water:
		🥛🥛🥛🥛 🥛🥛🥛🥛
		Sleep (Hours):
Proteins: ___ g Carbs: ___ g Fats: ___ g	Proteins: ___ g Carbs: ___ g Fats: ___ g	
DINNER	SNACKS	Exercise Type:
		_____
		Exercise (Minutes):
Proteins: ___ g Carbs: ___ g Fats: ___ g	Proteins: ___ g Carbs: ___ g Fats: ___ g	
DAILY MACROS Proteins: ___ % Carbs: ___ % Fats: ___ %		

Notes:

DAY 136 Date: _____ Mood Check: 😀 🙂 😐 🙁 ☹️

BREAKFAST	LUNCH	Water:
		🥛🥛🥛🥛 🥛🥛🥛🥛
		Sleep (Hours):
Proteins: ___ g Carbs: ___ g Fats: ___ g	Proteins: ___ g Carbs: ___ g Fats: ___ g	
DINNER	SNACKS	Exercise Type:
		_____
		Exercise (Minutes):
Proteins: ___ g Carbs: ___ g Fats: ___ g	Proteins: ___ g Carbs: ___ g Fats: ___ g	
DAILY MACROS Proteins: ___ % Carbs: ___ % Fats: ___ %		

Notes:

WEEK 20

DAY 137 Date: _____ Mood Check: 😀 🙂 😐 🙁 😞

BREAKFAST

Proteins: ___ g Carbs: ___ g Fats: ___ g

LUNCH

Proteins: ___ g Carbs: ___ g Fats: ___ g

Water:

Sleep (Hours):
_____

DINNER

Proteins: ___ g Carbs: ___ g Fats: ___ g

SNACKS

Proteins: ___ g Carbs: ___ g Fats: ___ g

Exercise Type:
_____

Exercise (Minutes):

DAILY MACROS   Proteins: ___ %   Carbs: ___ %   Fats: ___ %

Notes:

DAY 138 Date: _____ Mood Check: 😀 🙂 😐 🙁 😞

BREAKFAST

Proteins: ___ g Carbs: ___ g Fats: ___ g

LUNCH

Proteins: ___ g Carbs: ___ g Fats: ___ g

Water:

Sleep (Hours):
_____

DINNER

Proteins: ___ g Carbs: ___ g Fats: ___ g

SNACKS

Proteins: ___ g Carbs: ___ g Fats: ___ g

Exercise Type:
_____

Exercise (Minutes):

DAILY MACROS   Proteins: ___ %   Carbs: ___ %   Fats: ___ %

Notes:

DAY 139

Date: _____ Mood Check: 😀 🙂 😐 🙁 😣

BREAKFAST	LUNCH	Water:
		🥛🥛🥛🥛 🥛🥛🥛🥛
		Sleep (Hours):
Proteins: ___ g Carbs: ___ g Fats: ___ g	Proteins: ___ g Carbs: ___ g Fats: ___ g	_____
DINNER	**SNACKS**	Exercise Type: _____ Exercise (Minutes):
Proteins: ___ g Carbs: ___ g Fats: ___ g	Proteins: ___ g Carbs: ___ g Fats: ___ g	
DAILY MACROS Proteins: ___ % Carbs: ___ % Fats: ___ %		_____

Notes:

DAY 140

Date: _____ Mood Check: 😀 🙂 😐 🙁 😣

BREAKFAST	LUNCH	Water:
		🥛🥛🥛🥛 🥛🥛🥛🥛
		Sleep (Hours):
Proteins: ___ g Carbs: ___ g Fats: ___ g	Proteins: ___ g Carbs: ___ g Fats: ___ g	_____
DINNER	**SNACKS**	Exercise Type: _____ Exercise (Minutes):
Proteins: ___ g Carbs: ___ g Fats: ___ g	Proteins: ___ g Carbs: ___ g Fats: ___ g	
DAILY MACROS Proteins: ___ % Carbs: ___ % Fats: ___ %		_____

Notes:

FOUR-WEEK CHECK-IN

Date: _____

MEASUREMENT	CURRENT	MONTH CHANGE
WEIGHT (LB)		
UPPER ARMS (IN)		
CHEST (IN)		
WAIST (IN)		
HIPS (IN)		
THIGHS (IN)		
CALVES (IN)		

CONGRATULATIONS ON MAKING IT THIS FAR!

What are you most proud of accomplishing in the past four weeks?

_____

_____

_____

_____

What was your biggest challenge over the past four weeks?

_____

_____

_____

_____

_____

What are some goals you would like to work toward for the next four weeks?

_____

_____

_____

_____

Reflect on your mood over the past month. Did you notice differences related to your eating habits?

_____

_____

_____

_____

_____

WEEKLY INTENTION

What are you excited about for this week?

Proteins: _____ %
Carbs: _____ %
Fats: _____ %

_____

_____

_____

What is something you'd like to work on this week? _____

_____

_____

_____

DAY 141	Date: _____	Mood Check: 😃 🙂 😐 🙁 ☹️
BREAKFAST	**LUNCH**	Water:
		🥛🥛🥛🥛🥛 🥛🥛🥛🥛🥛
		Sleep (Hours):
Proteins: ___ g Carbs: ___ g Fats: ___ g	Proteins: ___ g Carbs: ___ g Fats: ___ g	_____
DINNER	**SNACKS**	Exercise Type:
		_____
		Exercise (Minutes):
Proteins: ___ g Carbs: ___ g Fats: ___ g	Proteins: ___ g Carbs: ___ g Fats: ___ g	_____
DAILY MACROS	Proteins: ___ % Carbs: ___ % Fats: ___ %	

Notes:

DAY 142

Date: _____ Mood Check: 😃 🙂 😐 🙁 😟

BREAKFAST	LUNCH	Water:
		🥤🥤🥤🥤 🥤🥤🥤🥤
		Sleep (Hours):
Proteins: ___ g Carbs: ___ g Fats: ___ g	Proteins: ___ g Carbs: ___ g Fats: ___ g	_____
DINNER	**SNACKS**	**Exercise Type:**
		_____
		Exercise (Minutes):
Proteins: ___ g Carbs: ___ g Fats: ___ g	Proteins: ___ g Carbs: ___ g Fats: ___ g	
DAILY MACROS Proteins: ___% Carbs: ___% Fats: ___%		_____

Notes:

DAY 143

Date: _____ Mood Check: 😃 🙂 😐 🙁 😟

BREAKFAST	LUNCH	Water:
		🥤🥤🥤🥤 🥤🥤🥤🥤
		Sleep (Hours):
Proteins: ___ g Carbs: ___ g Fats: ___ g	Proteins: ___ g Carbs: ___ g Fats: ___ g	_____
DINNER	**SNACKS**	**Exercise Type:**
		_____
		Exercise (Minutes):
Proteins: ___ g Carbs: ___ g Fats: ___ g	Proteins: ___ g Carbs: ___ g Fats: ___ g	
DAILY MACROS Proteins: ___% Carbs: ___% Fats: ___%		_____

Notes:

DAY 144 Date: _____ Mood Check: 😃 🙂 😐 🙁 ☹️

BREAKFAST	LUNCH	Water:
		🥤🥤🥤🥤 🥤🥤🥤🥤
		Sleep (Hours):
Proteins: ___ g Carbs: ___ g Fats: ___ g	Proteins: ___ g Carbs: ___ g Fats: ___ g	_____
DINNER	**SNACKS**	Exercise Type:
		_____
		Exercise (Minutes):
Proteins: ___ g Carbs: ___ g Fats: ___ g	Proteins: ___ g Carbs: ___ g Fats: ___ g	_____
DAILY MACROS Proteins: ___ % Carbs: ___ % Fats: ___ %		

Notes:

DAY 145 Date: _____ Mood Check: 😃 🙂 😐 🙁 ☹️

BREAKFAST	LUNCH	Water:
		🥤🥤🥤🥤 🥤🥤🥤🥤
		Sleep (Hours):
Proteins: ___ g Carbs: ___ g Fats: ___ g	Proteins: ___ g Carbs: ___ g Fats: ___ g	_____
DINNER	**SNACKS**	Exercise Type:
		_____
		Exercise (Minutes):
Proteins: ___ g Carbs: ___ g Fats: ___ g	Proteins: ___ g Carbs: ___ g Fats: ___ g	_____
DAILY MACROS Proteins: ___ % Carbs: ___ % Fats: ___ %		

Notes:

DAY 146 Date: _____ Mood Check: 😀 🙂 😐 🙁 ☹️

BREAKFAST	LUNCH	Water:
		🥛🥛🥛🥛🥛 🥛🥛🥛🥛🥛
		Sleep (Hours):
Proteins: ___ g Carbs: ___ g Fats: ___ g	Proteins: ___ g Carbs: ___ g Fats: ___ g	_____
DINNER	SNACKS	Exercise Type:
		_____
		Exercise (Minutes):
Proteins: ___ g Carbs: ___ g Fats: ___ g	Proteins: ___ g Carbs: ___ g Fats: ___ g	
DAILY MACROS Proteins: ___ % Carbs: ___ % Fats: ___ %		_____

Notes:

DAY 147 Date: _____ Mood Check: 😀 🙂 😐 🙁 ☹️

BREAKFAST	LUNCH	Water:
		🥛🥛🥛🥛🥛 🥛🥛🥛🥛🥛
		Sleep (Hours):
Proteins: ___ g Carbs: ___ g Fats: ___ g	Proteins: ___ g Carbs: ___ g Fats: ___ g	_____
DINNER	SNACKS	Exercise Type:
		_____
		Exercise (Minutes):
Proteins: ___ g Carbs: ___ g Fats: ___ g	Proteins: ___ g Carbs: ___ g Fats: ___ g	
DAILY MACROS Proteins: ___ % Carbs: ___ % Fats: ___ %		_____

Notes:

WEEKLY INTENTION

What are you excited about for this week?

_____

_____

_____

_____

What is something you'd like to work on this week? _____

_____

_____

_____

Proteins: _____ %
Carbs: _____ %
Fats: _____ %

DAY 148 Date: _____ Mood Check: 😊 🙂 😐 🙁 ☹️

BREAKFAST	LUNCH	Water:
		🥛🥛🥛🥛 🥛🥛🥛🥛
		Sleep (Hours):
Proteins: ___ g Carbs: ___ g Fats: ___ g	Proteins: ___ g Carbs: ___ g Fats: ___ g	_____
DINNER	SNACKS	Exercise Type:
		_____
		Exercise (Minutes):
Proteins: ___ g Carbs: ___ g Fats: ___ g	Proteins: ___ g Carbs: ___ g Fats: ___ g	
DAILY MACROS Proteins: ___ % Carbs: ___ % Fats: ___ %		_____

Notes:

DAY 149

Date: _____ Mood Check: 😃 🙂 😐 🙁 😞

BREAKFAST	LUNCH	Water:
		🥛🥛🥛🥛🥛 🥛🥛🥛🥛🥛
		Sleep (Hours):
Proteins: ___ g Carbs: ___ g Fats: ___ g	Proteins: ___ g Carbs: ___ g Fats: ___ g	_____
DINNER	**SNACKS**	Exercise Type:
		_____
		Exercise (Minutes):
Proteins: ___ g Carbs: ___ g Fats: ___ g	Proteins: ___ g Carbs: ___ g Fats: ___ g	
DAILY MACROS Proteins: ___ % Carbs: ___ % Fats: ___ %		_____

Notes:

DAY 150

Date: _____ Mood Check: 😃 🙂 😐 🙁 😞

BREAKFAST	LUNCH	Water:
		🥛🥛🥛🥛🥛 🥛🥛🥛🥛🥛
		Sleep (Hours):
Proteins: ___ g Carbs: ___ g Fats: ___ g	Proteins: ___ g Carbs: ___ g Fats: ___ g	_____
DINNER	**SNACKS**	Exercise Type:
		_____
		Exercise (Minutes):
Proteins: ___ g Carbs: ___ g Fats: ___ g	Proteins: ___ g Carbs: ___ g Fats: ___ g	
DAILY MACROS Proteins: ___ % Carbs: ___ % Fats: ___ %		_____

Notes:

DAY 151

Date: _____ Mood Check: 😃 😊 😐 🙁 😣

BREAKFAST	LUNCH	Water:
		🥛🥛🥛🥛🥛 🥛🥛🥛🥛🥛
		Sleep (Hours):
Proteins: ___ g Carbs: ___ g Fats: ___ g	Proteins: ___ g Carbs: ___ g Fats: ___ g	_____
DINNER	**SNACKS**	Exercise Type: _____ Exercise (Minutes):
Proteins: ___ g Carbs: ___ g Fats: ___ g	Proteins: ___ g Carbs: ___ g Fats: ___ g	
DAILY MACROS Proteins: ___ % Carbs: ___ % Fats: ___ %		

Notes:

DAY 152

Date: _____ Mood Check: 😃 😊 😐 🙁 😣

BREAKFAST	LUNCH	Water:
		🥛🥛🥛🥛🥛 🥛🥛🥛🥛🥛
		Sleep (Hours):
Proteins: ___ g Carbs: ___ g Fats: ___ g	Proteins: ___ g Carbs: ___ g Fats: ___ g	_____
DINNER	**SNACKS**	Exercise Type: _____ Exercise (Minutes):
Proteins: ___ g Carbs: ___ g Fats: ___ g	Proteins: ___ g Carbs: ___ g Fats: ___ g	
DAILY MACROS Proteins: ___ % Carbs: ___ % Fats: ___ %		

Notes:

DAY 153 Date: _____ Mood Check: 😊 🙂 😐 🙁 😞

BREAKFAST	LUNCH	Water:
		🥤🥤🥤🥤 🥤🥤🥤🥤
		Sleep (Hours):
Proteins: ___ g Carbs: ___ g Fats: ___ g	Proteins: ___ g Carbs: ___ g Fats: ___ g	
DINNER	SNACKS	Exercise Type:
		_____
		Exercise (Minutes):
Proteins: ___ g Carbs: ___ g Fats: ___ g	Proteins: ___ g Carbs: ___ g Fats: ___ g	
DAILY MACROS Proteins: ___ % Carbs: ___ % Fats: ___ %		

Notes:

DAY 154 Date: _____ Mood Check: 😊 🙂 😐 🙁 😞

BREAKFAST	LUNCH	Water:
		🥤🥤🥤🥤 🥤🥤🥤🥤
		Sleep (Hours):
Proteins: ___ g Carbs: ___ g Fats: ___ g	Proteins: ___ g Carbs: ___ g Fats: ___ g	
DINNER	SNACKS	Exercise Type:
		_____
		Exercise (Minutes):
Proteins: ___ g Carbs: ___ g Fats: ___ g	Proteins: ___ g Carbs: ___ g Fats: ___ g	
DAILY MACROS Proteins: ___ % Carbs: ___ % Fats: ___ %		

Notes:

WEEKLY INTENTION

What are you excited about for this week?

Proteins: _____ %
Carbs: _____ %
Fats: _____ %

_____

_____

_____

_____

What is something you'd like to work on this week? _____

_____

_____

_____

DAY 155	Date: _____	Mood Check: 😀 🙂 😐 🙁 ☹️
BREAKFAST	**LUNCH**	Water:
		Sleep (Hours):
Proteins: ___ g Carbs: ___ g Fats: ___ g	Proteins: ___ g Carbs: ___ g Fats: ___ g	_____
DINNER	**SNACKS**	Exercise Type:
		_____
		Exercise (Minutes):
Proteins: ___ g Carbs: ___ g Fats: ___ g	Proteins: ___ g Carbs: ___ g Fats: ___ g	
DAILY MACROS Proteins: ___% Carbs: ___% Fats: ___%		_____

Notes:

DAY 156

Date: _____ Mood Check: 😃 🙂 😐 🙁 ☹️

BREAKFAST

Proteins: ___ g Carbs: ___ g Fats: ___ g

LUNCH

Proteins: ___ g Carbs: ___ g Fats: ___ g

DINNER

Proteins: ___ g Carbs: ___ g Fats: ___ g

SNACKS

Proteins: ___ g Carbs: ___ g Fats: ___ g

DAILY MACROS   Proteins: ___ %   Carbs: ___ %   Fats: ___ %

Water:

Sleep (Hours): _____

Exercise Type: _____

Exercise (Minutes): _____

Notes:

DAY 157

Date: _____ Mood Check: 😃 🙂 😐 🙁 ☹️

BREAKFAST

Proteins: ___ g Carbs: ___ g Fats: ___ g

LUNCH

Proteins: ___ g Carbs: ___ g Fats: ___ g

DINNER

Proteins: ___ g Carbs: ___ g Fats: ___ g

SNACKS

Proteins: ___ g Carbs: ___ g Fats: ___ g

DAILY MACROS   Proteins: ___ %   Carbs: ___ %   Fats: ___ %

Water:

Sleep (Hours): _____

Exercise Type: _____

Exercise (Minutes): _____

Notes:

DAY 158 Date: _____ Mood Check: 😃 🙂 😐 🙁 😟

BREAKFAST	LUNCH	Water:
		🥛🥛🥛🥛 🥛🥛🥛🥛
		Sleep (Hours):
Proteins: ___ g Carbs: ___ g Fats: ___ g	Proteins: ___ g Carbs: ___ g Fats: ___ g	_____
DINNER	SNACKS	Exercise Type: _____
		Exercise (Minutes):
Proteins: ___ g Carbs: ___ g Fats: ___ g	Proteins: ___ g Carbs: ___ g Fats: ___ g	
DAILY MACROS Proteins: ___ % Carbs: ___ % Fats: ___ %		_____

Notes:

DAY 159 Date: _____ Mood Check: 😃 🙂 😐 🙁 😟

BREAKFAST	LUNCH	Water:
		🥛🥛🥛🥛 🥛🥛🥛🥛
		Sleep (Hours):
Proteins: ___ g Carbs: ___ g Fats: ___ g	Proteins: ___ g Carbs: ___ g Fats: ___ g	_____
DINNER	SNACKS	Exercise Type: _____
		Exercise (Minutes):
Proteins: ___ g Carbs: ___ g Fats: ___ g	Proteins: ___ g Carbs: ___ g Fats: ___ g	
DAILY MACROS Proteins: ___ % Carbs: ___ % Fats: ___ %		_____

Notes:

DAY 160

Date: _____ Mood Check: 😀 🙂 😐 🙁 ☹️

BREAKFAST	LUNCH	Water:
		🥤🥤🥤🥤 🥤🥤🥤🥤
		Sleep (Hours):
Proteins: ___ g Carbs: ___ g Fats: ___ g	Proteins: ___ g Carbs: ___ g Fats: ___ g	_____
DINNER	**SNACKS**	Exercise Type:
		_____
		Exercise (Minutes):
Proteins: ___ g Carbs: ___ g Fats: ___ g	Proteins: ___ g Carbs: ___ g Fats: ___ g	
DAILY MACROS Proteins: ___ % Carbs: ___ % Fats: ___ %		_____

Notes:

DAY 161

Date: _____ Mood Check: 😀 🙂 😐 🙁 ☹️

BREAKFAST	LUNCH	Water:
		🥤🥤🥤🥤 🥤🥤🥤🥤
		Sleep (Hours):
Proteins: ___ g Carbs: ___ g Fats: ___ g	Proteins: ___ g Carbs: ___ g Fats: ___ g	_____
DINNER	**SNACKS**	Exercise Type:
		_____
		Exercise (Minutes):
Proteins: ___ g Carbs: ___ g Fats: ___ g	Proteins: ___ g Carbs: ___ g Fats: ___ g	
DAILY MACROS Proteins: ___ % Carbs: ___ % Fats: ___ %		_____

Notes:

WEEKLY INTENTION

What are you excited about for this week?

Proteins: _____ %
Carbs: _____ %
Fats: _____ %

_____

_____

_____

What is something you'd like to work on this week? _____

_____

_____

_____

DAY 162	Date: _____	Mood Check: 😃 🙂 😐 🙁 ☹️
BREAKFAST	**LUNCH**	Water:
		Sleep (Hours):
Proteins: ___ g Carbs: ___ g Fats: ___ g	Proteins: ___ g Carbs: ___ g Fats: ___ g	_____
DINNER	**SNACKS**	Exercise Type: _____ Exercise (Minutes):
Proteins: ___ g Carbs: ___ g Fats: ___ g	Proteins: ___ g Carbs: ___ g Fats: ___ g	_____
DAILY MACROS Proteins: ___ % Carbs: ___ % Fats: ___ %		

Notes:

DAY 163   Date: _____   Mood Check: 😀 🙂 😐 🙁 😞

BREAKFAST	LUNCH	Water:
		🥛🥛🥛🥛 🥛🥛🥛🥛
		Sleep (Hours):
Proteins: ___ g Carbs: ___ g Fats: ___ g	Proteins: ___ g Carbs: ___ g Fats: ___ g	_____
DINNER	**SNACKS**	Exercise Type:
		_____
		Exercise (Minutes):
Proteins: ___ g Carbs: ___ g Fats: ___ g	Proteins: ___ g Carbs: ___ g Fats: ___ g	_____
DAILY MACROS Proteins: ___ % Carbs: ___ % Fats: ___ %		

Notes:

DAY 164   Date: _____   Mood Check: 😀 🙂 😐 🙁 😞

BREAKFAST	LUNCH	Water:
		🥛🥛🥛🥛 🥛🥛🥛🥛
		Sleep (Hours):
Proteins: ___ g Carbs: ___ g Fats: ___ g	Proteins: ___ g Carbs: ___ g Fats: ___ g	_____
DINNER	**SNACKS**	Exercise Type:
		_____
		Exercise (Minutes):
Proteins: ___ g Carbs: ___ g Fats: ___ g	Proteins: ___ g Carbs: ___ g Fats: ___ g	_____
DAILY MACROS Proteins: ___ % Carbs: ___ % Fats: ___ %		

Notes:

DAY 165

Date: _____ Mood Check: 😃 😊 😐 😟 😣

BREAKFAST	LUNCH	Water:
		Sleep (Hours):
Proteins: ___ g Carbs: ___ g Fats: ___ g	Proteins: ___ g Carbs: ___ g Fats: ___ g	_____
DINNER	SNACKS	Exercise Type:
		_____
		Exercise (Minutes):
Proteins: ___ g Carbs: ___ g Fats: ___ g	Proteins: ___ g Carbs: ___ g Fats: ___ g	
DAILY MACROS Proteins: ___ % Carbs: ___ % Fats: ___ %		

Notes:

DAY 166

Date: _____ Mood Check: 😃 😊 😐 😟 😣

BREAKFAST	LUNCH	Water:
		Sleep (Hours):
Proteins: ___ g Carbs: ___ g Fats: ___ g	Proteins: ___ g Carbs: ___ g Fats: ___ g	_____
DINNER	SNACKS	Exercise Type:
		_____
		Exercise (Minutes):
Proteins: ___ g Carbs: ___ g Fats: ___ g	Proteins: ___ g Carbs: ___ g Fats: ___ g	
DAILY MACROS Proteins: ___ % Carbs: ___ % Fats: ___ %		

Notes:

DAY 167   Date: _____   Mood Check: 😃 😊 😐 🙁 😣

BREAKFAST	LUNCH	Water:
		🥛🥛🥛🥛🥛 🥛🥛🥛🥛🥛
		Sleep (Hours):
Proteins: ___ g Carbs: ___ g Fats: ___ g	Proteins: ___ g Carbs: ___ g Fats: ___ g	_____
DINNER	SNACKS	Exercise Type: _____
		Exercise (Minutes):
Proteins: ___ g Carbs: ___ g Fats: ___ g	Proteins: ___ g Carbs: ___ g Fats: ___ g	_____
DAILY MACROS Proteins: ___ % Carbs: ___ % Fats: ___ %		

Notes:

DAY 168   Date: _____   Mood Check: 😃 😊 😐 🙁 😣

BREAKFAST	LUNCH	Water:
		🥛🥛🥛🥛🥛 🥛🥛🥛🥛🥛
		Sleep (Hours):
Proteins: ___ g Carbs: ___ g Fats: ___ g	Proteins: ___ g Carbs: ___ g Fats: ___ g	_____
DINNER	SNACKS	Exercise Type: _____
		Exercise (Minutes):
Proteins: ___ g Carbs: ___ g Fats: ___ g	Proteins: ___ g Carbs: ___ g Fats: ___ g	_____
DAILY MACROS Proteins: ___ % Carbs: ___ % Fats: ___ %		

Notes:

FOUR-WEEK CHECK-IN

Date: _____

MEASUREMENT	CURRENT	MONTH CHANGE
WEIGHT (LB)		
UPPER ARMS (IN)		
CHEST (IN)		
WAIST (IN)		
HIPS (IN)		
THIGHS (IN)		
CALVES (IN)		

CONGRATULATIONS ON MAKING IT THIS FAR!

What are you most proud of accomplishing in the past four weeks?

_____

_____

_____

_____

What was your biggest challenge over the past four weeks?

_____

_____

_____

_____

_____

What are some goals you would like to work toward for the next four weeks?

_____

_____

_____

_____

Reflect on your mood over the past month. Did you notice differences related to your eating habits?

_____

_____

_____

_____

_____

WEEK 25

WEEKLY INTENTION

TARGET MACROS

What are you excited about for this week?

Proteins: _____ %
Carbs: _____ %
Fats: _____ %

_____

_____

_____

What is something you'd like to work on this week? _____

_____

_____

_____

DAY 169	Date: _____	Mood Check: ☺ ☺ ☺ ☹ ☹
BREAKFAST	**LUNCH**	Water:
		🥛🥛🥛🥛🥛 🥛🥛🥛🥛🥛
		Sleep (Hours):
Proteins: ___ g Carbs: ___ g Fats: ___ g	Proteins: ___ g Carbs: ___ g Fats: ___ g	_____
DINNER	**SNACKS**	Exercise Type:
		_____
		Exercise (Minutes):
Proteins: ___ g Carbs: ___ g Fats: ___ g	Proteins: ___ g Carbs: ___ g Fats: ___ g	
DAILY MACROS	Proteins: ___ % Carbs: ___ % Fats: ___ %	_____

Notes:

DAY 170 Date: _____ Mood Check: 😃 🙂 😐 🙁 😞

BREAKFAST	LUNCH	Water:
		🥛🥛🥛🥛 🥛🥛🥛🥛
		Sleep (Hours):
Proteins: ___ g Carbs: ___ g Fats: ___ g	Proteins: ___ g Carbs: ___ g Fats: ___ g	_____

DINNER	SNACKS	Exercise Type:
		_____
		Exercise (Minutes):
Proteins: ___ g Carbs: ___ g Fats: ___ g	Proteins: ___ g Carbs: ___ g Fats: ___ g	_____

DAILY MACROS   Proteins: ___ %   Carbs: ___ %   Fats: ___ %

Notes:

DAY 171 Date: _____ Mood Check: 😃 🙂 😐 🙁 😞

BREAKFAST	LUNCH	Water:
		🥛🥛🥛🥛 🥛🥛🥛🥛
		Sleep (Hours):
Proteins: ___ g Carbs: ___ g Fats: ___ g	Proteins: ___ g Carbs: ___ g Fats: ___ g	_____

DINNER	SNACKS	Exercise Type:
		_____
		Exercise (Minutes):
Proteins: ___ g Carbs: ___ g Fats: ___ g	Proteins: ___ g Carbs: ___ g Fats: ___ g	_____

DAILY MACROS   Proteins: ___ %   Carbs: ___ %   Fats: ___ %

Notes:

WEEK 25

DAY 172   Date: _____   Mood Check: 😃 🙂 😐 🙁 ☹️

BREAKFAST	LUNCH	Water:
		🥛🥛🥛🥛 🥛🥛🥛🥛
		Sleep (Hours):
Proteins: ___ g Carbs: ___ g Fats: ___ g	Proteins: ___ g Carbs: ___ g Fats: ___ g	_____
DINNER	SNACKS	Exercise Type:
		_____
		Exercise (Minutes):
Proteins: ___ g Carbs: ___ g Fats: ___ g	Proteins: ___ g Carbs: ___ g Fats: ___ g	_____
DAILY MACROS Proteins: ___ % Carbs: ___ % Fats: ___ %		

Notes:

DAY 173   Date: _____   Mood Check: 😃 🙂 😐 🙁 ☹️

BREAKFAST	LUNCH	Water:
		🥛🥛🥛🥛 🥛🥛🥛🥛
		Sleep (Hours):
Proteins: ___ g Carbs: ___ g Fats: ___ g	Proteins: ___ g Carbs: ___ g Fats: ___ g	_____
DINNER	SNACKS	Exercise Type:
		_____
		Exercise (Minutes):
Proteins: ___ g Carbs: ___ g Fats: ___ g	Proteins: ___ g Carbs: ___ g Fats: ___ g	_____
DAILY MACROS Proteins: ___ % Carbs: ___ % Fats: ___ %		

Notes:

DAY 174 Date: _____ Mood Check: 😊 🙂 😐 🙁 😣

BREAKFAST	LUNCH	Water:
		🥤🥤🥤🥤🥤 🥤🥤🥤🥤🥤
		Sleep (Hours):
Proteins: ___ g Carbs: ___ g Fats: ___ g	Proteins: ___ g Carbs: ___ g Fats: ___ g	_____
DINNER	**SNACKS**	Exercise Type: _____ Exercise (Minutes):
Proteins: ___ g Carbs: ___ g Fats: ___ g	Proteins: ___ g Carbs: ___ g Fats: ___ g	
DAILY MACROS Proteins: ___% Carbs: ___% Fats: ___%		_____

Notes:

DAY 175 Date: _____ Mood Check: 😊 🙂 😐 🙁 😣

BREAKFAST	LUNCH	Water:
		🥤🥤🥤🥤🥤 🥤🥤🥤🥤🥤
		Sleep (Hours):
Proteins: ___ g Carbs: ___ g Fats: ___ g	Proteins: ___ g Carbs: ___ g Fats: ___ g	_____
DINNER	**SNACKS**	Exercise Type: _____ Exercise (Minutes):
Proteins: ___ g Carbs: ___ g Fats: ___ g	Proteins: ___ g Carbs: ___ g Fats: ___ g	
DAILY MACROS Proteins: ___% Carbs: ___% Fats: ___%		_____

Notes:

WEEKLY INTENTION

What are you excited about for this week?

Proteins: _____ %
Carbs: _____ %
Fats: _____ %

_____

_____

_____

_____

What is something you'd like to work on this week? _____

_____

_____

_____

DAY 176	Date: _____	Mood Check: 😀 🙂 😐 🙁 ☹️
BREAKFAST	**LUNCH**	Water:
		🥛🥛🥛🥛 🥛🥛🥛🥛
		Sleep (Hours):
Proteins: ___ g Carbs: ___ g Fats: ___ g	Proteins: ___ g Carbs: ___ g Fats: ___ g	_____
DINNER	**SNACKS**	Exercise Type:
		_____
		Exercise (Minutes):
Proteins: ___ g Carbs: ___ g Fats: ___ g	Proteins: ___ g Carbs: ___ g Fats: ___ g	_____
DAILY MACROS Proteins: ___ % Carbs: ___ % Fats: ___ %		

Notes:

DAY 177

Date: _____ Mood Check: 😀 🙂 😐 🙁 😣

BREAKFAST	LUNCH	Water:
		🥛🥛🥛🥛 🥛🥛🥛🥛
		Sleep (Hours):
Proteins: ___ g Carbs: ___ g Fats: ___ g	Proteins: ___ g Carbs: ___ g Fats: ___ g	_____
DINNER	SNACKS	Exercise Type:
		_____
		Exercise (Minutes):
Proteins: ___ g Carbs: ___ g Fats: ___ g	Proteins: ___ g Carbs: ___ g Fats: ___ g	
DAILY MACROS	Proteins: ___ % Carbs: ___ % Fats: ___ %	

Notes:

DAY 178

Date: _____ Mood Check: 😀 🙂 😐 🙁 😣

BREAKFAST	LUNCH	Water:
		🥛🥛🥛🥛 🥛🥛🥛🥛
		Sleep (Hours):
Proteins: ___ g Carbs: ___ g Fats: ___ g	Proteins: ___ g Carbs: ___ g Fats: ___ g	_____
DINNER	SNACKS	Exercise Type:
		_____
		Exercise (Minutes):
Proteins: ___ g Carbs: ___ g Fats: ___ g	Proteins: ___ g Carbs: ___ g Fats: ___ g	
DAILY MACROS	Proteins: ___ % Carbs: ___ % Fats: ___ %	

Notes:

DAY 179   Date: _____   Mood Check: 😃 🙂 😐 🙁 ☹️

BREAKFAST

Proteins: ___ g Carbs: ___ g Fats: ___ g

LUNCH

Proteins: ___ g Carbs: ___ g Fats: ___ g

Water:

Sleep (Hours):

_____

DINNER

Proteins: ___ g Carbs: ___ g Fats: ___ g

SNACKS

Proteins: ___ g Carbs: ___ g Fats: ___ g

Exercise Type:

_____

Exercise (Minutes):

DAILY MACROS   Proteins: ___ %   Carbs: ___ %   Fats: ___ %

_____

Notes:

DAY 180   Date: _____   Mood Check: 😃 🙂 😐 🙁 ☹️

BREAKFAST

Proteins: ___ g Carbs: ___ g Fats: ___ g

LUNCH

Proteins: ___ g Carbs: ___ g Fats: ___ g

Water:

Sleep (Hours):

_____

DINNER

Proteins: ___ g Carbs: ___ g Fats: ___ g

SNACKS

Proteins: ___ g Carbs: ___ g Fats: ___ g

Exercise Type:

_____

Exercise (Minutes):

DAILY MACROS   Proteins: ___ %   Carbs: ___ %   Fats: ___ %

_____

Notes:

DAY 181 | Date: _____ Mood Check: 😃 🙂 😐 🙁 😣

BREAKFAST	LUNCH	Water:
		🥤🥤🥤🥤 🥤🥤🥤🥤
		Sleep (Hours):
Proteins: ___ g Carbs: ___ g Fats: ___ g	Proteins: ___ g Carbs: ___ g Fats: ___ g	_____
DINNER	**SNACKS**	Exercise Type:
		_____
		Exercise (Minutes):
Proteins: ___ g Carbs: ___ g Fats: ___ g	Proteins: ___ g Carbs: ___ g Fats: ___ g	_____
DAILY MACROS Proteins: ___ % Carbs: ___ % Fats: ___ %		

Notes:

DAY 182 | Date: _____ Mood Check: 😃 🙂 😐 🙁 😣

BREAKFAST	LUNCH	Water:
		🥤🥤🥤🥤 🥤🥤🥤🥤
		Sleep (Hours):
Proteins: ___ g Carbs: ___ g Fats: ___ g	Proteins: ___ g Carbs: ___ g Fats: ___ g	_____
DINNER	**SNACKS**	Exercise Type:
		_____
		Exercise (Minutes):
Proteins: ___ g Carbs: ___ g Fats: ___ g	Proteins: ___ g Carbs: ___ g Fats: ___ g	_____
DAILY MACROS Proteins: ___ % Carbs: ___ % Fats: ___ %		

Notes:

WEEKLY INTENTION

What are you excited about for this week?

Proteins: _____ %
Carbs: _____ %
Fats: _____ %

_____

_____

_____

_____

What is something you'd like to work on this week? _____

_____

_____

_____

DAY 183	Date: _____	Mood Check: 😀 🙂 😐 🙁 😞

BREAKFAST	LUNCH	Water:
		🥛🥛🥛🥛🥛 🥛🥛🥛🥛🥛
		Sleep (Hours):
Proteins: ___g Carbs: ___g Fats: ___g	Proteins: ___g Carbs: ___g Fats: ___g	
DINNER	SNACKS	Exercise Type:
		Exercise (Minutes):
Proteins: ___g Carbs: ___g Fats: ___g	Proteins: ___g Carbs: ___g Fats: ___g	

DAILY MACROS   Proteins: ___%   Carbs: ___%   Fats: ___%

Notes:

DAY 184

Date: _____   Mood Check: 😀 🙂 😐 🙁 ☹️

BREAKFAST	LUNCH	Water:
		🥛🥛🥛🥛🥛
		🥛🥛🥛🥛🥛
		Sleep (Hours):
Proteins: ___ g Carbs: ___ g Fats: ___ g	Proteins: ___ g Carbs: ___ g Fats: ___ g	_____

DINNER	SNACKS	Exercise Type:
		_____
		Exercise (Minutes):
Proteins: ___ g Carbs: ___ g Fats: ___ g	Proteins: ___ g Carbs: ___ g Fats: ___ g	

DAILY MACROS   Proteins: ___ %   Carbs: ___ %   Fats: ___ %   _____

Notes:

DAY 185

Date: _____   Mood Check: 😀 🙂 😐 🙁 ☹️

BREAKFAST	LUNCH	Water:
		🥛🥛🥛🥛🥛
		🥛🥛🥛🥛🥛
		Sleep (Hours):
Proteins: ___ g Carbs: ___ g Fats: ___ g	Proteins: ___ g Carbs: ___ g Fats: ___ g	_____

DINNER	SNACKS	Exercise Type:
		_____
		Exercise (Minutes):
Proteins: ___ g Carbs: ___ g Fats: ___ g	Proteins: ___ g Carbs: ___ g Fats: ___ g	

DAILY MACROS   Proteins: ___ %   Carbs: ___ %   Fats: ___ %   _____

Notes:

DAY 186   Date: _____   Mood Check: 😃 🙂 😐 🙁 😦

BREAKFAST	LUNCH	Water:
		🥛🥛🥛🥛 🥛🥛🥛🥛
		Sleep (Hours):
Proteins: ___ g Carbs: ___ g Fats: ___ g	Proteins: ___ g Carbs: ___ g Fats: ___ g	_____
DINNER	SNACKS	Exercise Type:
		_____
		Exercise (Minutes):
Proteins: ___ g Carbs: ___ g Fats: ___ g	Proteins: ___ g Carbs: ___ g Fats: ___ g	_____
DAILY MACROS Proteins: ___ % Carbs: ___ % Fats: ___ %		

Notes:

DAY 187   Date: _____   Mood Check: 😃 🙂 😐 🙁 😦

BREAKFAST	LUNCH	Water:
		🥛🥛🥛🥛 🥛🥛🥛🥛
		Sleep (Hours):
Proteins: ___ g Carbs: ___ g Fats: ___ g	Proteins: ___ g Carbs: ___ g Fats: ___ g	_____
DINNER	SNACKS	Exercise Type:
		_____
		Exercise (Minutes):
Proteins: ___ g Carbs: ___ g Fats: ___ g	Proteins: ___ g Carbs: ___ g Fats: ___ g	_____
DAILY MACROS Proteins: ___ % Carbs: ___ % Fats: ___ %		

Notes:

DAY 188

Date: _____ Mood Check: 😀 🙂 😐 🙁 ☹️

BREAKFAST

Proteins: ___ g Carbs: ___ g Fats: ___ g

LUNCH

Proteins: ___ g Carbs: ___ g Fats: ___ g

DINNER

Proteins: ___ g Carbs: ___ g Fats: ___ g

SNACKS

Proteins: ___ g Carbs: ___ g Fats: ___ g

Water:

Sleep (Hours):
_____

Exercise Type:
_____

Exercise (Minutes):
_____

DAILY MACROS   Proteins: ___ %   Carbs: ___ %   Fats: ___ %

Notes:

DAY 189

Date: _____ Mood Check: 😀 🙂 😐 🙁 ☹️

BREAKFAST

Proteins: ___ g Carbs: ___ g Fats: ___ g

LUNCH

Proteins: ___ g Carbs: ___ g Fats: ___ g

DINNER

Proteins: ___ g Carbs: ___ g Fats: ___ g

SNACKS

Proteins: ___ g Carbs: ___ g Fats: ___ g

Water:

Sleep (Hours):
_____

Exercise Type:
_____

Exercise (Minutes):
_____

DAILY MACROS   Proteins: ___ %   Carbs: ___ %   Fats: ___ %

Notes:

WEEKLY INTENTION

What are you excited about for this week?

Proteins: _____ %
Carbs: _____ %
Fats: _____ %

_____

_____

_____

What is something you'd like to work on this week? _____

_____

_____

_____

DAY 190	Date: _____	Mood Check: ☺ ☺ ☺ ☹ ☹
BREAKFAST	**LUNCH**	Water:
		🥛🥛🥛🥛🥛 🥛🥛🥛🥛🥛
		Sleep (Hours):
Proteins: ___ g Carbs: ___ g Fats: ___ g	Proteins: ___ g Carbs: ___ g Fats: ___ g	_____
DINNER	**SNACKS**	Exercise Type:
		_____
		Exercise (Minutes):
Proteins: ___ g Carbs: ___ g Fats: ___ g	Proteins: ___ g Carbs: ___ g Fats: ___ g	_____
DAILY MACROS Proteins: ___ % Carbs: ___ % Fats: ___ %		

Notes:

DAY 191

Date: _____ Mood Check: 😀 ☺ 😐 🙁 ☹

BREAKFAST	LUNCH	Water:
		🥛🥛🥛🥛 🥛🥛🥛🥛
		Sleep (Hours):
Proteins: ___ g Carbs: ___ g Fats: ___ g	Proteins: ___ g Carbs: ___ g Fats: ___ g	_____
DINNER	**SNACKS**	Exercise Type:
		_____
		Exercise (Minutes):
Proteins: ___ g Carbs: ___ g Fats: ___ g	Proteins: ___ g Carbs: ___ g Fats: ___ g	
DAILY MACROS Proteins: ___ % Carbs: ___ % Fats: ___ %		_____

Notes:

DAY 192

Date: _____ Mood Check: 😀 ☺ 😐 🙁 ☹

BREAKFAST	LUNCH	Water:
		🥛🥛🥛🥛 🥛🥛🥛🥛
		Sleep (Hours):
Proteins: ___ g Carbs: ___ g Fats: ___ g	Proteins: ___ g Carbs: ___ g Fats: ___ g	_____
DINNER	**SNACKS**	Exercise Type:
		_____
		Exercise (Minutes):
Proteins: ___ g Carbs: ___ g Fats: ___ g	Proteins: ___ g Carbs: ___ g Fats: ___ g	
DAILY MACROS Proteins: ___ % Carbs: ___ % Fats: ___ %		_____

Notes:

DAY 193

Date: _____ Mood Check: 😃 😊 😐 😕 😣

BREAKFAST

LUNCH

Water:

Sleep (Hours):
_____

Proteins: ___ g Carbs: ___ g Fats: ___ g

Proteins: ___ g Carbs: ___ g Fats: ___ g

DINNER

SNACKS

Exercise Type:

_____

Exercise (Minutes):

Proteins: ___ g Carbs: ___ g Fats: ___ g

Proteins: ___ g Carbs: ___ g Fats: ___ g

DAILY MACROS   Proteins: ___ % Carbs: ___ % Fats: ___ %

_____

Notes:

DAY 194

Date: _____ Mood Check: 😃 😊 😐 😕 😣

BREAKFAST

LUNCH

Water:

Sleep (Hours):
_____

Proteins: ___ g Carbs: ___ g Fats: ___ g

Proteins: ___ g Carbs: ___ g Fats: ___ g

DINNER

SNACKS

Exercise Type:

_____

Exercise (Minutes):

Proteins: ___ g Carbs: ___ g Fats: ___ g

Proteins: ___ g Carbs: ___ g Fats: ___ g

DAILY MACROS   Proteins: ___ % Carbs: ___ % Fats: ___ %

_____

Notes:

DAY 195 Date: _____ Mood Check: ☺ ☺ ☺ ☺ ☹

BREAKFAST	LUNCH	Water:
		🥛🥛🥛🥛🥛 🥛🥛🥛🥛🥛
		Sleep (Hours):
Proteins: ___ g Carbs: ___ g Fats: ___ g	Proteins: ___ g Carbs: ___ g Fats: ___ g	_____
DINNER	SNACKS	Exercise Type:
		_____
		Exercise (Minutes):
Proteins: ___ g Carbs: ___ g Fats: ___ g	Proteins: ___ g Carbs: ___ g Fats: ___ g	
DAILY MACROS Proteins: ___ % Carbs: ___ % Fats: ___ %		

Notes:

DAY 196 Date: _____ Mood Check: ☺ ☺ ☺ ☺ ☹

BREAKFAST	LUNCH	Water:
		🥛🥛🥛🥛🥛 🥛🥛🥛🥛🥛
		Sleep (Hours):
Proteins: ___ g Carbs: ___ g Fats: ___ g	Proteins: ___ g Carbs: ___ g Fats: ___ g	_____
DINNER	SNACKS	Exercise Type:
		_____
		Exercise (Minutes):
Proteins: ___ g Carbs: ___ g Fats: ___ g	Proteins: ___ g Carbs: ___ g Fats: ___ g	
DAILY MACROS Proteins: ___ % Carbs: ___ % Fats: ___ %		

Notes:

FOUR-WEEK CHECK-IN

Date: _____

MEASUREMENT	CURRENT	MONTH CHANGE
WEIGHT (LB)		
UPPER ARMS (IN)		
CHEST (IN)		
WAIST (IN)		
HIPS (IN)		
THIGHS (IN)		
CALVES (IN)		

CONGRATULATIONS ON MAKING IT THIS FAR!

What are you most proud of accomplishing in the past four weeks?

_____

_____

_____

_____

What was your biggest challenge over the past four weeks?

_____

_____

_____

_____

_____

What are some goals you would like to work toward for the next four weeks?

_____

_____

_____

_____

_____

Reflect on your mood over the past month. Did you notice differences related to your eating habits?

_____

_____

_____

_____

_____

_____

WEEKLY INTENTION

What are you excited about for this week?

Proteins: _____ %
Carbs: _____ %
Fats: _____ %

_____

_____

_____

What is something you'd like to work on this week? _____

_____

_____

_____

DAY 197	Date: _____	Mood Check: 😃 😊 😐 🙁 ☹️
BREAKFAST	**LUNCH**	Water:
		🥛🥛🥛🥛🥛 🥛🥛🥛🥛🥛
		Sleep (Hours):
Proteins: ___ g Carbs: ___ g Fats: ___ g	Proteins: ___ g Carbs: ___ g Fats: ___ g	_____
DINNER	**SNACKS**	Exercise Type:
		_____
		Exercise (Minutes):
Proteins: ___ g Carbs: ___ g Fats: ___ g	Proteins: ___ g Carbs: ___ g Fats: ___ g	
DAILY MACROS Proteins: ___ % Carbs: ___ % Fats: ___ %		_____

Notes:

DAY 198 Date: _____ Mood Check: 😀 🙂 😐 🙁 😞

BREAKFAST	LUNCH	Water:
		🥛🥛🥛🥛 🥛🥛🥛🥛
		Sleep (Hours):
Proteins: ___ g Carbs: ___ g Fats: ___ g	Proteins: ___ g Carbs: ___ g Fats: ___ g	_____
DINNER	SNACKS	Exercise Type:
		_____
		Exercise (Minutes):
Proteins: ___ g Carbs: ___ g Fats: ___ g	Proteins: ___ g Carbs: ___ g Fats: ___ g	
DAILY MACROS Proteins: ___ % Carbs: ___ % Fats: ___ %		_____

Notes:

DAY 199 Date: _____ Mood Check: 😀 🙂 😐 🙁 😞

BREAKFAST	LUNCH	Water:
		🥛🥛🥛🥛 🥛🥛🥛🥛
		Sleep (Hours):
Proteins: ___ g Carbs: ___ g Fats: ___ g	Proteins: ___ g Carbs: ___ g Fats: ___ g	_____
DINNER	SNACKS	Exercise Type:
		_____
		Exercise (Minutes):
Proteins: ___ g Carbs: ___ g Fats: ___ g	Proteins: ___ g Carbs: ___ g Fats: ___ g	
DAILY MACROS Proteins: ___ % Carbs: ___ % Fats: ___ %		_____

Notes:

DAY 200   Date: _____   Mood Check: 😃 🙂 😐 🙁 😣

BREAKFAST	LUNCH	Water:
		🥤🥤🥤🥤🥤 🥤🥤🥤🥤🥤
		Sleep (Hours):
Proteins: ___ g Carbs: ___ g Fats: ___ g	Proteins: ___ g Carbs: ___ g Fats: ___ g	_____
DINNER	SNACKS	Exercise Type:
		_____
		Exercise (Minutes):
Proteins: ___ g Carbs: ___ g Fats: ___ g	Proteins: ___ g Carbs: ___ g Fats: ___ g	
DAILY MACROS Proteins: ___ % Carbs: ___ % Fats: ___ %		_____

Notes:

DAY 201   Date: _____   Mood Check: 😃 🙂 😐 🙁 😣

BREAKFAST	LUNCH	Water:
		🥤🥤🥤🥤🥤 🥤🥤🥤🥤🥤
		Sleep (Hours):
Proteins: ___ g Carbs: ___ g Fats: ___ g	Proteins: ___ g Carbs: ___ g Fats: ___ g	_____
DINNER	SNACKS	Exercise Type:
		_____
		Exercise (Minutes):
Proteins: ___ g Carbs: ___ g Fats: ___ g	Proteins: ___ g Carbs: ___ g Fats: ___ g	
DAILY MACROS Proteins: ___ % Carbs: ___ % Fats: ___ %		_____

Notes:

DAY 202 Date: _____ Mood Check: 😀 🙂 😐 🙁 😞

BREAKFAST	LUNCH	Water:
		🥛🥛🥛🥛 🥛🥛🥛🥛
		Sleep (Hours):
Proteins: ___ g Carbs: ___ g Fats: ___ g	Proteins: ___ g Carbs: ___ g Fats: ___ g	_____
DINNER	SNACKS	Exercise Type:
		_____
		Exercise (Minutes):
Proteins: ___ g Carbs: ___ g Fats: ___ g	Proteins: ___ g Carbs: ___ g Fats: ___ g	
DAILY MACROS Proteins: ___ % Carbs: ___ % Fats: ___ %		_____

Notes:

DAY 203 Date: _____ Mood Check: 😀 🙂 😐 🙁 😞

BREAKFAST	LUNCH	Water:
		🥛🥛🥛🥛 🥛🥛🥛🥛
		Sleep (Hours):
Proteins: ___ g Carbs: ___ g Fats: ___ g	Proteins: ___ g Carbs: ___ g Fats: ___ g	_____
DINNER	SNACKS	Exercise Type:
		_____
		Exercise (Minutes):
Proteins: ___ g Carbs: ___ g Fats: ___ g	Proteins: ___ g Carbs: ___ g Fats: ___ g	
DAILY MACROS Proteins: ___ % Carbs: ___ % Fats: ___ %		_____

Notes:

WEEKLY INTENTION

What are you excited about for this week?

_____

_____

_____

_____

What is something you'd like to work on this week? _____

_____

_____

_____

TARGET MACROS

Proteins: _____ %
Carbs: _____ %
Fats: _____ %

DAY 204	Date: _____	Mood Check: 😃 🙂 😐 😕 🙁

BREAKFAST	**LUNCH**	Water:
		🥛🥛🥛🥛 🥛🥛🥛🥛
		Sleep (Hours):
Proteins: ___ g Carbs: ___ g Fats: ___ g	Proteins: ___ g Carbs: ___ g Fats: ___ g	_____
DINNER	**SNACKS**	Exercise Type: _____
		Exercise (Minutes):
Proteins: ___ g Carbs: ___ g Fats: ___ g	Proteins: ___ g Carbs: ___ g Fats: ___ g	_____

DAILY MACROS   Proteins: ___%   Carbs: ___%   Fats: ___%

Notes:

DAY 205   Date: _____   Mood Check: 😀 ☺ 😐 🙁 ☹

BREAKFAST	LUNCH	Water:
		🥛🥛🥛🥛 🥛🥛🥛🥛
		Sleep (Hours):
Proteins: ___ g Carbs: ___ g Fats: ___ g	Proteins: ___ g Carbs: ___ g Fats: ___ g	_____
DINNER	**SNACKS**	Exercise Type:
		_____
		Exercise (Minutes):
Proteins: ___ g Carbs: ___ g Fats: ___ g	Proteins: ___ g Carbs: ___ g Fats: ___ g	_____
DAILY MACROS Proteins: ___ % Carbs: ___ % Fats: ___ %		

Notes:

DAY 206   Date: _____   Mood Check: 😀 ☺ 😐 🙁 ☹

BREAKFAST	LUNCH	Water:
		🥛🥛🥛🥛 🥛🥛🥛🥛
		Sleep (Hours):
Proteins: ___ g Carbs: ___ g Fats: ___ g	Proteins: ___ g Carbs: ___ g Fats: ___ g	_____
DINNER	**SNACKS**	Exercise Type:
		_____
		Exercise (Minutes):
Proteins: ___ g Carbs: ___ g Fats: ___ g	Proteins: ___ g Carbs: ___ g Fats: ___ g	_____
DAILY MACROS Proteins: ___ % Carbs: ___ % Fats: ___ %		

Notes:

DAY 207

Date: _____   Mood Check: 😀 🙂 😐 🙁 ☹️

BREAKFAST

Proteins: ___ g Carbs: ___ g Fats: ___ g

LUNCH

Proteins: ___ g Carbs: ___ g Fats: ___ g

Water:

Sleep (Hours):

_____

DINNER

Proteins: ___ g Carbs: ___ g Fats: ___ g

SNACKS

Proteins: ___ g Carbs: ___ g Fats: ___ g

Exercise Type:

_____

Exercise (Minutes):

_____

DAILY MACROS   Proteins: ___ %   Carbs: ___ %   Fats: ___ %

Notes:

DAY 208

Date: _____   Mood Check: 😀 🙂 😐 🙁 ☹️

BREAKFAST

Proteins: ___ g Carbs: ___ g Fats: ___ g

LUNCH

Proteins: ___ g Carbs: ___ g Fats: ___ g

Water:

Sleep (Hours):

_____

DINNER

Proteins: ___ g Carbs: ___ g Fats: ___ g

SNACKS

Proteins: ___ g Carbs: ___ g Fats: ___ g

Exercise Type:

_____

Exercise (Minutes):

_____

DAILY MACROS   Proteins: ___ %   Carbs: ___ %   Fats: ___ %

Notes:

DAY 209   Date: _____   Mood Check: 😀 ☺ 😐 ☹ 😣

BREAKFAST	LUNCH	Water:
		🥛🥛🥛🥛 🥛🥛🥛🥛
		Sleep (Hours):
Proteins: ___ g Carbs: ___ g Fats: ___ g	Proteins: ___ g Carbs: ___ g Fats: ___ g	_____
DINNER	SNACKS	Exercise Type:
		_____
		Exercise (Minutes):
Proteins: ___ g Carbs: ___ g Fats: ___ g	Proteins: ___ g Carbs: ___ g Fats: ___ g	
DAILY MACROS Proteins: ___ % Carbs: ___ % Fats: ___ %		_____

Notes:

DAY 210   Date: _____   Mood Check: 😀 ☺ 😐 ☹ 😣

BREAKFAST	LUNCH	Water:
		🥛🥛🥛🥛 🥛🥛🥛🥛
		Sleep (Hours):
Proteins: ___ g Carbs: ___ g Fats: ___ g	Proteins: ___ g Carbs: ___ g Fats: ___ g	_____
DINNER	SNACKS	Exercise Type:
		_____
		Exercise (Minutes):
Proteins: ___ g Carbs: ___ g Fats: ___ g	Proteins: ___ g Carbs: ___ g Fats: ___ g	
DAILY MACROS Proteins: ___ % Carbs: ___ % Fats: ___ %		_____

Notes:

WEEKLY INTENTION

What are you excited about for this week?

Proteins: _____ %
Carbs: _____ %
Fats: _____ %

_____

_____

_____

_____

What is something you'd like to work on this week? _____

_____

_____

_____

DAY 211	Date: _____	Mood Check: 😃 🙂 😐 🙁 😢
BREAKFAST	**LUNCH**	Water:
		Sleep (Hours):
Proteins: ___ g Carbs: ___ g Fats: ___ g	Proteins: ___ g Carbs: ___ g Fats: ___ g	_____
DINNER	**SNACKS**	Exercise Type: _____
		Exercise (Minutes):
Proteins: ___ g Carbs: ___ g Fats: ___ g	Proteins: ___ g Carbs: ___ g Fats: ___ g	_____
DAILY MACROS Proteins: ___ % Carbs: ___ % Fats: ___ %		

Notes:

DAY 212
Date: _____ Mood Check: 😄 🙂 😐 🙁 😣

BREAKFAST

LUNCH

Water:

🥛 🥛 🥛 🥛 🥛
🥛 🥛 🥛 🥛 🥛

Sleep (Hours):

Proteins: ___ g Carbs: ___ g Fats: ___ g

Proteins: ___ g Carbs: ___ g Fats: ___ g

_____

DINNER

SNACKS

Exercise
Type:

_____

Exercise
(Minutes):

Proteins: ___ g Carbs: ___ g Fats: ___ g

Proteins: ___ g Carbs: ___ g Fats: ___ g

DAILY MACROS Proteins: ___ % Carbs: ___ % Fats: ___ %

_____

Notes:

DAY 213
Date: _____ Mood Check: 😄 🙂 😐 🙁 😣

BREAKFAST

LUNCH

Water:

🥛 🥛 🥛 🥛 🥛
🥛 🥛 🥛 🥛 🥛

Sleep (Hours):

Proteins: ___ g Carbs: ___ g Fats: ___ g

Proteins: ___ g Carbs: ___ g Fats: ___ g

_____

DINNER

SNACKS

Exercise
Type:

_____

Exercise
(Minutes):

Proteins: ___ g Carbs: ___ g Fats: ___ g

Proteins: ___ g Carbs: ___ g Fats: ___ g

DAILY MACROS Proteins: ___ % Carbs: ___ % Fats: ___ %

_____

Notes:

DAY 214   Date: _____   Mood Check: 😃 🙂 😐 🙁 😣

BREAKFAST	LUNCH	Water:
		🥛🥛🥛🥛 🥛🥛🥛🥛
		Sleep (Hours):
Proteins: ___ g Carbs: ___ g Fats: ___ g	Proteins: ___ g Carbs: ___ g Fats: ___ g	_____
DINNER	**SNACKS**	Exercise Type:
		_____
		Exercise (Minutes):
Proteins: ___ g Carbs: ___ g Fats: ___ g	Proteins: ___ g Carbs: ___ g Fats: ___ g	_____
DAILY MACROS Proteins: ___ % Carbs: ___ % Fats: ___ %		

Notes:

DAY 215   Date: _____   Mood Check: 😃 🙂 😐 🙁 😣

BREAKFAST	LUNCH	Water:
		🥛🥛🥛🥛 🥛🥛🥛🥛
		Sleep (Hours):
Proteins: ___ g Carbs: ___ g Fats: ___ g	Proteins: ___ g Carbs: ___ g Fats: ___ g	_____
DINNER	**SNACKS**	Exercise Type:
		_____
		Exercise (Minutes):
Proteins: ___ g Carbs: ___ g Fats: ___ g	Proteins: ___ g Carbs: ___ g Fats: ___ g	_____
DAILY MACROS Proteins: ___ % Carbs: ___ % Fats: ___ %		

Notes:

DAY 216   Date: _____   Mood Check: 😃 ☺ 😐 🙁 ☹

BREAKFAST

LUNCH

Water:

Sleep (Hours):

_____

Proteins: ___ g   Carbs: ___ g   Fats: ___ g   Proteins: ___ g   Carbs: ___ g   Fats: ___ g

DINNER

SNACKS

Exercise Type:

_____

Exercise (Minutes):

Proteins: ___ g   Carbs: ___ g   Fats: ___ g   Proteins: ___ g   Carbs: ___ g   Fats: ___ g

DAILY MACROS   Proteins: ___%   Carbs: ___%   Fats: ___%

_____

Notes:

DAY 217   Date: _____   Mood Check: 😃 ☺ 😐 🙁 ☹

BREAKFAST

LUNCH

Water:

Sleep (Hours):

_____

Proteins: ___ g   Carbs: ___ g   Fats: ___ g   Proteins: ___ g   Carbs: ___ g   Fats: ___ g

DINNER

SNACKS

Exercise Type:

_____

Exercise (Minutes):

Proteins: ___ g   Carbs: ___ g   Fats: ___ g   Proteins: ___ g   Carbs: ___ g   Fats: ___ g

DAILY MACROS   Proteins: ___%   Carbs: ___%   Fats: ___%

_____

Notes:

WEEKLY INTENTION

What are you excited about for this week?

Proteins: _____ %
Carbs: _____ %
Fats: _____ %

_____

_____

_____

What is something you'd like to work on this week? _____

_____

_____

_____

DAY 218	Date: _____	Mood Check: ☺ ☺ ☺ ☹ ☹
BREAKFAST	**LUNCH**	Water:
		🥛🥛🥛🥛🥛 🥛🥛🥛🥛🥛
		Sleep (Hours):
Proteins: ___ g Carbs: ___ g Fats: ___ g	Proteins: ___ g Carbs: ___ g Fats: ___ g	_____
DINNER	**SNACKS**	Exercise Type:
		_____
		Exercise (Minutes):
Proteins: ___ g Carbs: ___ g Fats: ___ g	Proteins: ___ g Carbs: ___ g Fats: ___ g	
DAILY MACROS Proteins: ___ % Carbs: ___ % Fats: ___ %		_____

Notes:

DAY 219   Date: _____   Mood Check: 😃 🙂 😐 🙁 😣

BREAKFAST	LUNCH	Water:
		🥤🥤🥤🥤 🥤🥤🥤🥤
		Sleep (Hours):
Proteins: ___ g Carbs: ___ g Fats: ___ g	Proteins: ___ g Carbs: ___ g Fats: ___ g	_____
DINNER	**SNACKS**	Exercise Type:
		_____
		Exercise (Minutes):
Proteins: ___ g Carbs: ___ g Fats: ___ g	Proteins: ___ g Carbs: ___ g Fats: ___ g	
DAILY MACROS Proteins: ___ % Carbs: ___ % Fats: ___ %		_____

Notes:

DAY 220   Date: _____   Mood Check: 😃 🙂 😐 🙁 😣

BREAKFAST	LUNCH	Water:
		🥤🥤🥤🥤 🥤🥤🥤🥤
		Sleep (Hours):
Proteins: ___ g Carbs: ___ g Fats: ___ g	Proteins: ___ g Carbs: ___ g Fats: ___ g	_____
DINNER	**SNACKS**	Exercise Type:
		_____
		Exercise (Minutes):
Proteins: ___ g Carbs: ___ g Fats: ___ g	Proteins: ___ g Carbs: ___ g Fats: ___ g	
DAILY MACROS Proteins: ___ % Carbs: ___ % Fats: ___ %		_____

Notes:

DAY 221 Date: _____ Mood Check: 😀 🙂 😐 🙁 ☹️

BREAKFAST	LUNCH	Water:
		🥛🥛🥛🥛🥛 🥛🥛🥛🥛🥛
		Sleep (Hours):
Proteins: ___ g Carbs: ___ g Fats: ___ g	Proteins: ___ g Carbs: ___ g Fats: ___ g	_____
DINNER	SNACKS	Exercise Type:
		_____
		Exercise (Minutes):
Proteins: ___ g Carbs: ___ g Fats: ___ g	Proteins: ___ g Carbs: ___ g Fats: ___ g	_____
DAILY MACROS Proteins: ___ % Carbs: ___ % Fats: ___ %		

Notes:

DAY 222 Date: _____ Mood Check: 😀 🙂 😐 🙁 ☹️

BREAKFAST	LUNCH	Water:
		🥛🥛🥛🥛🥛 🥛🥛🥛🥛🥛
		Sleep (Hours):
Proteins: ___ g Carbs: ___ g Fats: ___ g	Proteins: ___ g Carbs: ___ g Fats: ___ g	_____
DINNER	SNACKS	Exercise Type:
		_____
		Exercise (Minutes):
Proteins: ___ g Carbs: ___ g Fats: ___ g	Proteins: ___ g Carbs: ___ g Fats: ___ g	_____
DAILY MACROS Proteins: ___ % Carbs: ___ % Fats: ___ %		

Notes:

DAY 223   Date: _____   Mood Check: 😃 🙂 😐 🙁 ☹️

BREAKFAST	LUNCH	Water:
		🥛🥛🥛🥛🥛 🥛🥛🥛🥛🥛
Proteins: ___ g Carbs: ___ g Fats: ___ g	Proteins: ___ g Carbs: ___ g Fats: ___ g	Sleep (Hours): _____
DINNER	SNACKS	Exercise Type: _____
		Exercise (Minutes):
Proteins: ___ g Carbs: ___ g Fats: ___ g	Proteins: ___ g Carbs: ___ g Fats: ___ g	_____

DAILY MACROS   Proteins: ___%   Carbs: ___%   Fats: ___%

Notes:

DAY 224   Date: _____   Mood Check: 😃 🙂 😐 🙁 ☹️

BREAKFAST	LUNCH	Water:
		🥛🥛🥛🥛🥛 🥛🥛🥛🥛🥛
Proteins: ___ g Carbs: ___ g Fats: ___ g	Proteins: ___ g Carbs: ___ g Fats: ___ g	Sleep (Hours): _____
DINNER	SNACKS	Exercise Type: _____
		Exercise (Minutes):
Proteins: ___ g Carbs: ___ g Fats: ___ g	Proteins: ___ g Carbs: ___ g Fats: ___ g	_____

DAILY MACROS   Proteins: ___%   Carbs: ___%   Fats: ___%

Notes:

FOUR-WEEK CHECK-IN

Date: _____

MEASUREMENT	CURRENT	MONTH CHANGE
WEIGHT (LB)		
UPPER ARMS (IN)		
CHEST (IN)		
WAIST (IN)		
HIPS (IN)		
THIGHS (IN)		
CALVES (IN)		

CONGRATULATIONS ON MAKING IT THIS FAR!

What are you most proud of accomplishing in the past four weeks?

_____

_____

_____

_____

What was your biggest challenge over the past four weeks?

_____

_____

_____

_____

_____

What are some goals you would like to work toward for the next four weeks?

_____

_____

_____

_____

_____

Reflect on your mood over the past month. Did you notice differences related to your eating habits?

_____

_____

_____

_____

_____

CPSIA information can be obtained
at www.ICGtesting.com
Printed in the USA
JSHW021916290422
25418JS00001B/2